The Secret History of a Woman Patient

Janet Rhys Dent

T0178957

Radcliffe Publishing
Oxford • Seattle

Radcliffe Publishing Ltd
18 Marcham Road
Abingdon
Oxon OX14 1AA
United Kingdom

www.radcliffe-oxford.com
Electronic catalogue and worldwide online ordering facility.

———————————————————

© 2007 Janet Rhys Dent

All rights reserved. No part of this publication may be reproduced, stored in a retrieval system or transmitted, in any form or by any means, electronic, mechanical, photocopying, recording or otherwise without the prior permission of the copyright owner.

Janet Rhys Dent has asserted her right under the Copyright, Designs and Patents Act, 1998, to be identified as Author of this Work.

Neither the publisher nor the authors accept liability for any injury or damage arising from this publication.

British Library Cataloguing in Publication Data

A catalogue record for this book is available from the British Library.

ISBN-10   1 84619 150 5
ISBN-13   978 184619 150 3

Typeset by Lapiz Digital Services, Chennai
Printed and bound by TJ International Ltd, Padstow, Cornwall

Contents

About the Author

Janet Rhys Dent grew up in Cymmer Afan and Port Talbot, South Wales. A former English Literature lecturer and researcher into diversity issues, she now lives and writes in the English Midlands where, following on from her membership of a Community Health Council, she works as a lay member of a Medical Research Ethics committee. Despite her work and training in the objective assessment of medical issues, she admits that after her diagnosis with breast cancer she morphed into a new patient who was by turns terrified, intrigued, intimidated, and inspired by the world of illness and medical treatment. These experiences continue to inform her life and work: she is the author of articles relating to ethical issues in medicine and education, and she conducts occasional workshops in creative writing that include the art of the memoir, journaling, and other forms of personal writing.

Acknowledgements

Deepest gratitude to all the women whose unrecorded stories have touched and inspired me, and most of all to my friend, Daphne Gick.

I am indebted to Bethan Lloyd Owen and other members of my medical team for their skills, knowledge and sustenance.

The poem, *Prognosis*, copyright 2005 by the Estate of Jane Kenyon, is reprinted from *Collected Poems* with the permission of Graywolf Press, Saint Paul, Minnesota, and with my thanks to Donald Hall, US Poet Laureate and husband of the late Jane Kenyon, for his kind help.

Thanks to Rhian Dent, not only for her encouragement but also for her delicacy and intelligence when it came to commenting on my manuscript as its pages slowly accumulated.

Professional and sincere gratitude to Gillian Nineham, editorial director of Radcliffe Publishing and to Gregory Moxon, Paula Jales and Lisa Abbott.

Fondest thanks to James and Sophie Dent; Elizabeth Davies; Freddie Gick; Judith Bevan; and, above all, to Tom, for faith, love and stalwart support.

Introduction

A few months after finishing my cancer treatment, I put in a request to look at my hospital medical notes. They duly arrived in the post in a flat A4 brown envelope. When I browsed through them, I was struck by the contrast between their bare facts and the breadth and depth of what had actually happened to me during the six-month period of my treatment. I had originally hoped, naively enough, for a report that gave me some new insight into my experience. But my medical notes were just a linear, chronological record of temperature, blood pressure and other measurable variables.

There was no indication of the fears, the hopes and the dilemmas that had been such an overwhelming part of my experience as a patient, and no hint of the challenges I faced both inside and outside the hospital during the critical period of my treatment. It was a time when I was clearly a patient in other people's eyes, but inside I was still trying to come to terms with this new identity and trying to work out how to be a patient. For the first time I realised that my life as a patient had been a silent, secret one as far as the medical staff and most of the other people with whom I came into contact were concerned.

This book depicts the secret life and the kind of survival strategies and decision-making processes that are a part of every woman's rite of passage as a patient. My book is based on the diary that I kept throughout my medical treatment, as well as on the knowledge that I have acquired in the five years since my illness. During this time I have gained insights through reflecting on my experiences, talking to other women patients and researching the works of theorists and writers, and through my experience and training as a voluntary worker in the NHS – as a lay member of a medical research ethics committee and a member of a community health council.

At times during my illness I viewed myself through the eyes of the medical staff, as an object – 'she', a passive, one-dimensional patient to be 'treated' – and one of the motives for writing this book was to redress the balance, to record the secret underworld of my time as a patient.

Although names and personal details have been changed in order to maintain confidentiality, all of the episodes in the book are true, real-life events. I portray the new world into which I am thrown, the search for knowledge about it, the people I meet, my attempts to understand and trust the hospital staff, system and treatment, and my failures and successes in adapting to many other challenges both outside and inside the hospital.

In particular, this is the story of my partly doomed quest to be a good patient so that fate would allow me to return to my old self and my old life after finishing my treatment. What is a good patient? What should one do? How should one act? How should one be in order to live as a good patient? My quest is itself a kind of survival strategy, and in pursuit of it I seek help from my family and friends, a support group called Bosom Friends, writers and theorists, Gaia (who was my Internet muse) and a variety of sources of self-help.

I record the kind of wild and stormy learning experience that never makes it into the medical notes, but that my fellow women patients might recognise. During the first months of medical tests, consultations, diagnosis, prognosis and treatment, women patients experience many congruent life-changing events and challenges. For example, when a serious illness comes along, how do you cope with your fear? How do you retain your identity as a woman, a mother, a partner, a colleague or any of the other identities of your everyday life? How do you relate to your family, friends, acquaintances and colleagues? How do you find out information about your illness and what is happening to you? How do you relate to the many medical professionals you meet, and the different kinds of medical settings in which you find yourself? How do you cope with mystifying medical procedures and with anticipated and unanticipated changes to your body? Can a support group help you? What happens when your treatment goes wrong?

When I look back at the period of my treatment for cancer, it's easy to identify dilemmas like these and it's even possible to detect a shape and a purpose to the way in which I grappled with them. But at the time everything seemed confusing, as I fell more and more into the role of patient and found myself having to continually let go of that 'me' who I thought I was, and my life as I knew it.

Why was it then that first one and then other women who were diagnosed with serious illness said 'It was one of the best things that ever happened to me'? Why would a life-threatening illness produce such a strong affirmation?

In the course of time, I came to know the answer to this question because I felt the same way. Of course we wished that we had never lost our health and that we did not have to face up to the new way of life that serious illness brings, with all of its fears and suffering. This is the life that others see, where women may be brave or fearful, but either way our experience may be viewed by others as exclusively negative and lonely. Yet all the while for so many women there is another secret life going on in which, despite our inevitable fears, we begin to see the world through another prism and its possibilities start to open out before us.

I found that it was a time when the concept of what it is to be a 'good patient' gradually began to lose the passive associations that it had once had for me and took on a new meaning as active and dynamic. I learned that life-threatening illness is not just a bodily event which leaves one's mind and identity unaltered, but a body–mind event, a time of inevitable change, when one may begin to move towards new self-understanding and begin to glimpse new possibilities of connection with others. And I learned that the essence of being a good patient was both simpler and more life-affirming than I had ever imagined.

CHAPTER 1

Discovery

I would never have expected trouble to strike then. Not in the sleepy Sunday twilight and not while I was slumped on my blue-striped sofa, unwinding after a busy day. A summer breeze drifted through the open window of my living room and its sudden coolness made me shiver. My warm fingers brushed across the skin just above the low neckline of my red cotton top, only to feel a small lump resisting their path. I paused, and then felt for the lump again. This time there was nothing there, just smooth skin over smooth flesh.

A few minutes later something made me try again and this time I found it. It seemed to be fixed in place. It couldn't be pushed around within my flesh, either from side to side or up and down. It wasn't soft and pliable like a fatty lump, but pebble-hard. It was an entity of its own and it felt alien. Fear clouded around my body, separating me from the rest of the room.

My book fell to the floor as I grabbed Paul's arm.

'Paul, I've found a lump.'

'A lump of what?'

'I've found a lump, just here, under my finger.'

He reached for the remote control and switched off the sound of the speeding car on the small screen.

'See if you can feel it.' I guided his index finger to the lump at the top of my right breast.

He palpated the lump in an objective kind of way, just as if I was one of his patients.

'Yes, there is a lump', he said. He took my hand. He'd not even gone back to watching his motoring programme. He's a GP, a family doctor. He usually looks at his own family's symptoms with the caution of one familiar with fly-by-night ailments: 'A bad cough? Breathe steam and see if it's better tomorrow.'

Now he said 'It's probably a cyst ... just harmless ... a benign cyst. Most breast lumps are cysts.'

I stared at the flickering television screen. Of course it was a cyst. Of course it was benign. Certainly not cancer. My body had a track record of good health and had managed to breastfeed three babies, although admittedly in a supplementary bottle-feeds and jars-of-chicken-broth sort of way. Moreover, I came from a long-living line of strong Welsh women, and it was my birthright to be healthy. My grandmothers lived until their late eighties, each free of disease until the final illness. My mother was 83, living in South Wales, and still fighting fit. This lump had to be a cyst – otherwise life was picking on me.

I wished I hadn't told Paul about the lump. Just by speaking about it, I'd given it a life of its own. I should have just forgotten about it. But it was already too late for that. Thoughts of illness and hospitals – in relation to other people's experiences as well as my own – were already racing through my mind. There was Sarah, a colleague at the college where I worked, who after treatment for a life-threatening heart condition had been in perfect health for the past 12 years. There was Meera, mother of two little schoolmates of my own two children, who'd been diagnosed with cervical cancer one December, and died just four months later. And then there was Emma, artist and close friend, who'd been diagnosed with cancer the previous year, soon after we had returned from an Easter trip to Venice. Now, a year later, she was fully recovered.

These memories were a jumble of feelings and images but very few facts. During the course of my life I'd absorbed ideas about illness from my family and other people, from stuff I'd read and films and television programmes I'd watched, but when it came to the medical facts, I'd acquired the idea that medical knowledge was exclusively for doctors to use, in whatever ways they thought best. Even working as a voluntary member of my local community health council hadn't changed my mindset. I'd contributed to basic research into patient satisfaction with various local hospital services, and gained some insight into the sometimes fraught relationships between patients and medical staff. Despite this training in the concept of the patient as an entitled consumer, deep down I still had the feeling that medical treatment was something that was done to the grateful patient by those who had expert knowledge.

Maybe this was why I had no memories of the medical facts of my friends' illnesses. They had been ill and had had treatment, but the rationale for it all was a mystery because it lay in the hands of the medical gods, nothing to do with the layperson.

It was the same with my memories of my own experiences as a patient. My hand compulsively prodded my lump as my mind flicked back to the time when I was a child and had my appendix removed. After the pain of my illness and my operation were eventually over, I had known that my recovery was down to my doctor, Dr Khan. Tall, young and witty, he'd appeared at my bedside as a nurse was about to give me an injection. Smiling into my unblinking eyes, he'd held my rigid hand. His casual orders to the nurses had indicated the confidence of one who was high up the hierarchical chain, and confirmed for me his godlike status. After that, whenever it was time for one of my four-hourly injections, I'd begged the nurses to fetch him so that he could hold my hand. He'd appeared on cue a couple of times, just often enough for me to feel sure that it was he and the expert grip of his strong, cool hands that were responsible for my healing.

In my twenties I was in and out of hospital for the delivery of each of my three children in turn, each time expecting the doctors to take the leading role in the delivery of my baby. Although I was not ill, I was in hospital and fell instinctively into the role of ignorant, trusting patient.

By the time of the birth of my first child, I had married a hospital doctor, my very own version of Dr Khan, hero of my childhood illness. Paul, a former house officer and then registrar, had been inducted into the hospital system and so, indirectly, had I. The hospital, with its medical staff and medical technology, was the natural place to go for a successful medical outcome, and the unspoken contract, it seemed to me, included a stipulation that the patient should surrender responsibility for treatment to the hospital staff.

All of these experiences from my own past now gave me the hope that any 'bio-extradition', whether it involved a baby, an appendix or a cancerous part of the body, would lead to a successful outcome – just so long as the procedure was devised and managed by medical staff. By this reasoning, removing the cancerous lump that lay rigid under my hand would mean the end of the cancer.

I even had nature's example of this – the potted palm with spiky green leaves that sat in my kitchen. Every time I watered it, I pulled lightly on the odd few spikes that had turned brown, and they fell away from the trunk. It was a satisfying ritual that had kept the plant healthy over many years. Yes, the human body is a lot more complex – but doctors have got science and technology on their side.

But what about women like Linda McCartney? Despite previous good health, a vegetarian diet and a happy family life, despite a successful career, and marriage to Paul McCartney, a venerated Beatle, despite a mastectomy and the best and most costly medical treatment, she died while she was still in her fifties. I brushed off this reminder of the limitations of medical science. I was a healthy person and had nothing to worry about.

The morning after I had discovered the lump, I awoke to blue sky and gentle rays of sunshine that wended their way through the branches of the pine tree outside our bedroom window. It was going to be another perfect summer's day. Then I remembered the lump. I forced myself to feel for it, hoping that it had all been a mistake. It was still there. Still in my pyjamas, I headed for the spare bedroom that I used as my study, although now it seemed like my court of appeal. Filled with an anxious sense of the future, waiting, I opened one of the windows and stared down at the avenue of blossom trees that watched over our suburban street. The only sound was the usual distant rumble of early-morning traffic leaving the peace of the countryside and suburbs and heading for Birmingham city centre, eight miles away.

I sat at the computer ready for the first time ever to seek information about a disease. Desperate for confirmation that my symptom was harmless and that I could carry on with my life as normal, I entered the address of my favourite search engine, which I'd named 'Gaia' after the Greek goddess of the earth. Gaia had helped me many times in the past. She'd found me an exercise bike, advised me on the rival merits of brick paving and tarmac when we needed a new front drive, and filled me in on the statistics relating to local schools.

Thanks to Gaia I felt more in control of the world because, although I might be a stranger to an area of knowledge, I could often surf my way to getting some kind of a grip on it. I didn't need to know the names of any medical experts or books or journals. Gaia would find suitable sites and put my mind at rest.

I typed 'breast cancer + cyst' into the search box, and then clicked on to one of the first of the ensuing list of related sites. It was that of an approved US medical college, so probably accurate, although I had learned from bitter experience to double-check useful information on other reputable sites.

I wanted to find out whether my lump was cancerous. The site described a benign, non-cancerous kind of breast lump called a cyst. I really, really wanted my lump to be a cyst. I learned that a cyst is filled with fluid. It is smooth and rubbery and, although it can feel tense and tender, it is mobile – it moves within the tissues. My heart sank – that wasn't my lump.

Another American site, a charity, told me that there are three kinds of lumps, two of which are benign. First, there is a cyst. Secondly, there is a fibroadenoma, which is a smooth rubbery lump that moves easily within the breast. The third kind, a breast tumour, is a hard lump that may or may not be tender and doesn't move easily. I was certain that my lump was neither of the first two, but I didn't want it to be the third one either. So the next question was whether there was any kind of breast lump that was hard and immobile, yet not cancerous. I typed 'breast cancer + hard lump' into the search box. I spent a further half hour looking through sites that were increasingly remote from my search term.

By now I'd forgotten that tumours are diagnosed with caution by doctors and only after thorough scientific analysis and assessment. By now, all of the information had merged in my mind into a single quest. I was desperate to find a description of a stony, immobile breast lump that was benign. I failed to find one.

Then once more I rallied. The Internet wasn't comprehensive, and vital information could be missing. Anyway, I probably lacked the skills to access the right kind of information. There was no proof that I had anything to worry about.

Downstairs, Paul was already sitting by the kitchen table, his grey-speckled black hair still glistening wet from his shower. He was eating toast spread with tinned tomatoes and cod liver oil. Tinned tomatoes had recently been shown to be healthier than fresh ones, and cod liver oil, since it was an effective food supplement, might just as well be incorporated into the daily menu. He pointed to an article on the front page of the *Guardian*, and said 'They're at it again. They're planning yet more changes for general practice ... it's a political football ...'.

I sat opposite him, my finger prodding the lump. One of the facts that I had learned from Gaia passed through my mind. Over 60% of cancerous lumps occur in the upper, outer quadrant of the breast. Just like mine.

In the past, Gaia had always given me the information that I required. Now I realised that all of that information had also been the information that I had wished for, that I actively wanted. What was on at the local cinema? Where could I track down a book on twentieth-century British film music? The answers had matched my expectations and left me feeling in charge of the whole data search. Now Gaia had begun to give me data about my lump that were unwelcome, even though this was information that I had sought.

Gaia was only a search engine, but I had been thinking of her as on my side. Now I saw that the Gaia who was my friend and my possession, who lived in my spare bedroom and gave me the requisite information to deal with the outside world – *that* Gaia was a myth. Gaia, goddess of the earth, actually *was* the outside world. Of course she was. She was impersonal and autonomous.

Paul seemed to have forgotten all about the lump. Was this a good sign? When it comes to breast lumps, GPs are used to being the bearers of good news, as nine out of ten of these lumps turn out to be benign. Part of me wanted to believe he was saying nothing because he was sure that my lump wasn't cancerous.

Suddenly I felt elated because the realisation hit me that I had the option of forgetting about the whole thing. Nothing and nobody could force me to do anything about my small, secret lump. I could just decide that it wasn't cancerous. It was in my power. It was my life after all. I felt relieved and excited by the prospect of just carrying on with my normal life.

Paul was still talking. 'And now the health authority wants to get rid of the protective screens in front of the receptionists. Violence in the surgery's getting increasingly common. Let's hope that the receptionists don't get hurt ...'.

That set me worrying about the receptionists in the health centre – Holly, Elaine and the others – and the way in which their security was being compromised.

It occurred to me that since I was worrying about other people in the outside world, my own worry must surely be trivial. Other things, much more important and much more devastating, were happening to other people all over the world.

As I loaded the white china breakfast bowls into the dishwasher, I stared at the dark lumps of congealed cereal that clung to them, wrecking their pure, clean shapes. These lumps were going to be removed by the dishwasher and its chemicals, leaving the dishes pure and sterilised. Yet I was thinking about conserving my unwanted lump, despite the fact that it might be not only waste matter but also dangerous matter.

'I'm off now', Paul said, putting on his jacket.

'Do you remember the lump I found?'

'Of course I do. You're worried about it, aren't you?'

'Do you think I should have it examined?'

'Yes. I'll make an appointment for you to have some tests at Rushwood Hospital as soon as possible', he said.

'Excellent. I'd like to get it all over with as soon as possible.'

'I'm sure everything will be fine. It's 90% likely to be benign.'

He gave me a quick kiss and hurried out of the kitchen, then paused to look back at me, his tall, bulky frame filling the doorway.

'See you later. Try not to worry.'

Alone in the kitchen, I stared at the picture on the front page of the newspaper showing a smiling Prince William, chin on hand, looking uncannily like his late mother, Princess Diana.

The lump must be benign. What a calming word, 'benign.' I associated it with fathers, priests and doctors. Men, not women, for some reason. Men with power who choose to use it kindly. Since it is used as the opposite of 'cancerous', cancerous must mean 'non-benign.' If benign was male, did that make non-benign female?

Non-benign, non-good, malevolent, full of bad. I couldn't identify any part of my body with those terms. My bodily systems, my vital organs, my cells – I'd always had the luxury of taking their benevolence towards me for granted. But now maybe I had cells in my body that were not benign, that were malignant. My body might be at war with itself, good cells against bad.

But how could I view my own cancer cells as malignant when they were mine? They didn't have any will of their own – they couldn't decide to be malignant or harmful. They were just cells. It was depressing to think that my body might be in conflict and that I might be involved in a fight with elements within it.

New as I was to cancer talk, I was using its everyday language of combat without realising that military terms were not in fact intrinsically related to cancer. I would later find, thanks both to the insights of theorists like Susan Sontag, in her book *Illness as Metaphor*, and to my own experiences, that cancer is in fact compatible with living a peaceful civilian life and that the battle imagery is optional. Thinking in terms of 'war' and 'good' and 'bad' isn't the only way to think of cancer.

Then words that my grandmother used to say – words that had always comforted me when I was a child – came into my mind: 'What happens is for the best.' Although I didn't understand what this strange kind of stoicism meant, and as I had grown older it had seemed simplistic, it had given a mystic sense of inevitability and reassurance to childhood losses like a missing doll or a briefly broken friendship. Later on in my life, long after my grandmother had died, bits and pieces of popular philosophy that I came across in books and newspapers at last gave me some insight into her thinking and the teachings of spiritual leaders like Julian of Norwich who had influenced her. The gist of it was that even the most painful aspects of reality may be celebrated as an occasion of joy if one learns to accept what happens as a gift. 'What happens is for the best.' Now part of me responded to these words, even as another part rejected them. No, there was no need for acceptance, no need because it involved recognising my symptom as a real threat, and it wasn't. It was just a benign lump.

I decided to get on with my day and put all worries about the lump out of my mind. Although the summer vacation had just started at the college where I worked as a part-time lecturer, I was due at a departmental meeting. Best to get on with life as normal. Things just couldn't change so quickly. Only the previous day everything had been normal.

There was nothing wrong with me. The aura of health still surrounded me and there was no way that I could suddenly turn into a patient, an ill person – not just like that.

I didn't realise, as I stepped out of the house for my college meeting, that my rite of passage as a patient had already started. Ironically, even in my frantic desire to forget about the symptom and all of its implications, I was already moving my stance on the world, already changing and taking on the role of patient.

Medical sociologists differentiate between illness and sickness. Sickness is the biological reality, whereas illness is what patients, families and doctors make of sickness. Illness, as Grimes points out in his book *Deeply into the Bone*, is how we frame and imagine sickness. That is what I was beginning to do. I was trying to work out what this potential sickness – cancer – might mean to me. I was engrossed in my own unique crisis and I was seeing it in my own personal and local terms, too wrapped up in my fears to realise that every day countless other women all over the world, in diverse circumstances and with diverse fears, face the same situation.

At that point all I could do was relate the significance of my lump to my previous health and that of my family, as well as to the experiences of friends. I looked back on the women I knew with cancer, as well as famous women like singer Carly Simon or writer Carole Shield, who I didn't know but whose encounters with cancer were in the public domain. I tried to remember what happened to them, and how other people regarded them. I was searching for clues and examples, and in doing so I was glimpsing what might lie in the future and preparing unknowingly for a separation from my present existence into a different stage of my life, a secret one, where I would begin to learn how to be a patient, how to relate to others as a patient, and how to live as a patient.

CHAPTER 2

Testing

'Samira Khan', called a nurse. The woman sitting opposite me jammed her feet back into her stilettos and followed the nurse into one of the adjoining consulting rooms. Just three days after I'd first discovered the lump in my breast, I was sitting in the smartly curtained and carpeted waiting room of Rushwood Hospital. I'd opted for the popular route of an initial outpatient consultation in a private hospital, with any necessary treatment taking place in our local National Health Service (NHS) hospital.

In her haste to get up, the woman opposite had dropped her magazine and, full of nervous energy, I sprang to retrieve it. It was a copy of *Yachting World*, and my gaze rested for a moment on the cover picture of a gleaming white cruiser escaping out to sea.

Someone sank into the seat next to me. It was Paul, newly arrived from his early evening surgery. How relieved I was to see his familiar face – someone who knew my life and was on my side – in that impersonal institution. He went to fetch two cups of water from the water cooler, and as he sat down again he noticed the name of my consultant on a nearby door.

'Would you like me to come in with you to see the consultant?'

'Yes, I would, thanks. But ... I think first of all I'd like to talk to him on my own, if you don't mind. Then I'll give you a shout.'

I wanted to avoid being cast in the role of 'doctor's wife' by the consultant, and the best way to do this was to visit him unaccompanied by a doctor husband. Far from attracting the preferential treatment that people often imagine, the role only seems to confuse. Whether in the hospital mess or in the health centre common room, I'd heard medics make remarks along the lines of 'Things always go wrong when it's a doctor's wife.' Neither doctors' husbands nor the live-in partners (male or female) of doctors seemed to attract this verdict, only doctors' wives. The woman referred to might have suffered an unlucky medical or surgical complication, but the inference was that she had colluded with misfortune in some way. I wanted to avoid any possibility of being stereotyped and have the consultant's attention focus on me as another routine, vulnerable patient.

Inside the consulting room, a heavily built man in his forties with a mop of brown curly hair rose from his oak desk to shake my hand. He gave me a small smile over the top of his half-moon gold spectacles, and then gestured towards an upholstered seat.

'Take a pew.'

As soon as I had sat down he asked, 'Now then, when exactly was it you discovered this lump?'

This seemed the perfect opportunity to give him the necessary information so that he could understand the nuances of what had happened to me so far.

I started my story. 'I was sitting on the sofa ...'

The consultant looked up, 'The date ...?'

I told him and then carried on, 'I came across a small lump ...'

He looked up again, put the top of his pen in his mouth and sighed.

'Could you please just answer my questions?'

I answered his brief list of questions with the required brief answers, but I was disappointed. The consultant had taken over my story and was fitting it into a format that he already knew but I didn't. There might be some aspect of my story that his questions wouldn't touch on but which might turn out to be significant. I had lost control of my story and now it was just a series of facts that made sense to him but not to me. I didn't know his sense and he didn't know mine.

Looking back, I'm aware that this was the first time I encountered what Foucault in *Birth of a Clinic* calls 'the medical gaze.' Foucault explores the ways in which the doctor has the power of science to see the hidden truth. This wisdom is acquired not from books but through the doctor's observation of patients. It is a practical wisdom learned through internships and apprenticeships. There is no way for anyone to challenge the doctor's experience because it just is.

Now, in the twenty-first century, I myself was intimidated by that medical gaze. My consultant had such wide experience and knowledge of other cases like mine, had been authenticated by a respected medical school and was now an expert authority at the top of the hospital hierarchy. It would be arrogant of me to claim any expertise with regard to my body. In the past I had automatically ceded all knowledge about my body to the doctor, but this time it was different. This lump was my lump not only because it was in my body, but also because I was the one who had found it. I knew its story so far and I clung to the details of it even as I recognised the consultant's supremacy and his potential to be my salvation.

It was a discord that I, like so many other women patients before me, would come across again and again:

> the tension between the power of the clinical gaze to diagnose and define breast cancer and the simultaneous construction of that knowledge by women through embodied and other knowledge sources.
>
> (Jennifer Fosket, *Problematising Biomedicine*)

Later on, I was to be the subject of further medical interrogations which would confirm that the medical staff were now the owners of my illness story. What is more, they were experts at whittling it down to what they considered to be its bare essentials. As time went on, if staff wanted to check a detail in my story they would look not at me but at my medical notes.

It would all make me realise how optimistic I had been at this early stage in expecting to take the lead in imparting my story. Spontaneous information from the patient was unwelcome, although questions were permissible as part of the patient's deferential role. I soon learned to speak only in response to the consultant's questions, and to bear in mind the limited time available for my consultation.

The consultant carried on with his questions: 'Is there any serious illness that runs in your family?'

'Nobody in my family has had cancer before', I said quickly. 'No one has ever had it, not on my mother's side or my father's side, not even a distant relative as far as I know.'

It was as if I was wheedling someone who had the power to block the threat of cancer, the implication being 'Please don't classify me. I'm not the usual cancer suspect, so please tell me that this cancer scare is a false alarm.'

The consultant showed no reaction. I later came across the statistic with which he was already familiar – 87% of women with breast cancer have no affected first-degree relatives (mother, sister or daughter), and many of them come from cancer-free families.

'Hop on the couch and I'll take a look', the consultant said.

Afterwards, I called Paul in to hear the consultant's verdict.

'Well, the lump doesn't seem to have the properties of a cancerous one. But I'd like you to have a mammogram and ultrasound just to be sure. We can do them straight away this evening.'

In the changing room, I draped a thin cotton hospital gown around my body in preparation for the mammogram, feeling as if I was becoming trapped in the world of illness even though I wasn't ill.

Samira Khan was already seated in the waiting area wearing an identical pink floral gown. She patted the chair next to her.

'Hi', she said. 'Sit here. Have you come for a check-up?'

'No. I've found a lump. I don't think it's cancer but I thought I'd better get it checked out ... just in case.'

'I hope it's not cancer. But if it is, it's not as bad as you probably think. I had breast cancer four years ago and this is my annual check-up.'

'You've been all right since?'

'Yes. I had chemotherapy. My hair fell out. I had to wear a wig. It was so itchy I decided to make myself a velvet bandana instead. It was quite smart, but it was also soft and cosy. When I didn't need it anymore, I made this hair band out of it. Now I always wear it when I'm coming for a check-up. It brings me luck.'

Her hand patted the blue and red striped velvet that glowed against her glossy black hair.

'I've been completely healthy ever since. The staff here have been very good ... and whenever I've needed it, I've had a lot of help from Bosom Friends, my support group.'

She rested her hand on my arm and looked at me. 'Sometimes I think my cancer was the best thing that ever happened to me. I'm a different person now to the one I used to be.'

'Oh ... right.'

I looked away, embarrassed. How could any woman ever think that having cancer was a good thing, let alone the best thing that had ever happened to her? I was sure that if I was diagnosed with cancer I would hate it, fight it and certainly never learn to accept it.

After Samira had gone, I sat breathing deeply in an attempt to calm the solid anxiety in my stomach. Pass or fail, this mammogram was a test that allowed no opportunity for practise or revision. Since the moment I had discovered my lump, I'd been at the centre of discussions about it. Now my lump was going to be tested and I had to be just a silent witness to the procedure. The lump that had been my own private discovery was now a public, clinical lump, outside my control.

'Can you slip your right arm out of your gown? Now stand here and push yourself as close as you can to the machine.'

Helen, with her long wavy hair and pink suede boots, looked reassuringly human for someone who was going to operate impersonal machinery.

She guided me into position. The tall, thin mammogram machine had an X-ray arm that reached about eight feet from the floor. In the middle were adjustable plates with armrests on each side. She placed me in a standing position and manoeuvred me into the pose that was necessary to ensure maximum exposure of flesh to the X-ray.

'Can you move a bit closer to the machine?'

I took two small steps.

'Great. Now lean to the right slightly.'

Helen hurried over to the controls to release me as soon as each X-ray, one for each side, had fired.

When it was all over, I sighed with relief. On to the next test, the ultrasound. 'Hang on a minute while I check these', said Helen. 'They might need redoing.'

Ten minutes later she was back. 'That's fine.'

'Could you see anything unusual in the X-rays?' I asked.

She shook her head. 'Sorry, I'm not allowed to give you any results. I'm just a technician. They'll let you know soon one way or another.'

Helen was a highly trained professional, but she was constrained by tiers of power and influence and banned from using her judgement and knowledge to give patients any information. What she saw on the X-ray films must be filtered through the 'team' that would be dealing with my case.

With a small shock I realised that I, the patient, was at the bottom of this hierarchy with no status and little power, and would be the last to know the verdict on my X-rays.

After the discomfort of the mammogram, the ultrasound was comparatively restful, the 'good-guy' interrogator of suspect lumps. The technician passed the sensor – what he called the ultrasound transducer – across the whole of my chest area in order to image any of those round and fluid-filled pockets known as cysts. If my lump was a cyst, that would be good news. The sensor could also quickly assess whether a suspicious area contained an increased density of solid tissue – the hard, dense mass that would signify bad news. I knew this because Gaia, my Internet muse, had told me.

The consultant arrived as the technician was finishing. I lay on the examination couch, my upper body propped up. I was now redundant. The required medical images were on the computer, and the two men stared at the ultrasound image on the screen.

'It's a hard lump', the technician told the consultant. My heart sank and I sighed loudly.

He ignored me. Unaware of the ranks of ordinary Web surfers like myself who, for good or ill, would relate what he said to what they had read on the Internet, he assumed that he was talking unfathomable medical jargon. My lump was hard. It was almost definitely not a cyst. I felt bitter disappointment but showed no outward reaction. Trapped once again in my passive patient role, I was reluctant to show knowledge of something that had not been officially imparted by a medical professional.

But then it occurred to me that the presence of two experts was too good an opportunity to miss. I had only been going on what I'd read on the Internet after all. It was a quixotic source compared with the verdict of two expert practitioners.

'Does the fact that it's a hard lump mean that it's a tumour?'

They both turned their heads to look at me.

Then the consultant said 'Nothing to worry about, at the moment. We'll be looking at the test results and then coming to a conclusion.'

'OK ... thanks.'

I gave up on my hopes of acquiring some information. I would have to wait for the usual formal procedure to run its course. Only then would the staff decree when and how much information I should be given.

The consultant said to me 'Some time next week I'd like to do a biopsy at Parkside Hospital.' Parkside was our local NHS hospital.

'You'll have a local anaesthetic to numb the area and then I'll take a small bit of tissue from the lump to test it.'

Scary as the tests had been, the fact that I had to have yet another one came as a relief. My fate was still in limbo. I was not a patient, just a normal person who was having some medical tests.

The long wait for the results of my tests began. I found myself worrying about the fact that I might die early, but at the same time I was letting my life slip by while I did it. Obsessed, I surfed the Web for facts, figures and findings about cancer, I scanned the sites of cancer charities, medical research institutes and hospitals, and I read the Internet blogs of women who had survived it and the posthumous ones of one or two who had died from it.

Sometimes I just sat in front of the computer, mutely staring at the screen, half lost. The reality of my future life seemed to lie there somewhere below the surface of the computer screen, just waiting to appear if only I could identify the right sequence of Internet sites and fully understand their contents.

I wondered whether I was now a patient. I had undergone medical tests at Rushwood Hospital. My lump had been biopsied at Parkside Hospital, where a needle had been inserted into the lump in order to harvest some of the cells. My details were being recorded on my medical records and I had an appointment to see the consultant in two weeks' time. All of this medical attention and yet I might turn out to be completely healthy.

In his book *The Limits of Medicine*, Illich says that '[testing] transforms people who feel healthy into patients feeling anxious for their verdict.' Then he goes on to pose two questions – whether you are only *not* a patient if you have been recently scrutinised by the medical profession, or whether health is a deeper and richer concept.

According to what I had learned from Gaia, my lump, if cancerous, could have been in my body for up to two years previously. During those years I had felt healthy and was living a healthy life. So had I been ill or healthy then?

I thought of a dinner party that had taken place when Emma, grey-faced and listless, was midway through her chemotherapy.

'I've always been naturally healthy', said Julie, our hostess. 'Colds and viruses and other nasty things just pass me by for some reason.'

Emma had been eating her tomato soup, but now put down her spoon and stared down in silence at the liquid in her bowl.

'None of us know what's going on in our bodies. None of us know for certain whether we are healthy. We could be harbouring symptoms at this very minute and not know it.' I said this as an act of solidarity, despite being utterly confident that I myself was completely healthy at that moment.

That conversation had taken place just a few months before I discovered my symptom, and I might have been harbouring a cancerous lump even as I spoke. No wonder that as I sat in front of my computer screen, the concept of health seemed more obscure than I had ever imagined it to be. If only I could stop my compulsive surfing. If my test results were bad news, I would be cast into the world of illness soon enough.

I was due to visit my mother in South Wales, and rang her to tell her about my lump. Slightly deaf, she enunciated down the phone in her usual energetic manner, 'Most breast lumps turn out to be nothing. Don't worry. You haven't got breast cancer. You can't have. You've never had very big breasts.'

I understood what she meant. As the only other female in a household with a father, three brothers and a charismatic, flirty mother, I was low down the woman stakes and, out of all the illnesses that might strike, certainly never destined for a womanly disease like breast cancer. My mother cited the number of friends she knew whose breast lumps had turned out to be benign, and when I visited her a few days later she invited one of them, Gwyneth, a solicitor, over for a cup of tea. We sat in my mother's deep pink and cream sitting room, surrounded by family photographs, including some of my late father. He had been headteacher of the town's comprehensive school, and my brothers, Gwyneth and I had all been his pupils.

After a few minutes my mother said, looking at Gwyneth, 'Well, I'll leave you now while I go and make the tea. Gwyneth's going to tell you about her breast lumps.'

My mother turned to me. Still good looking with clear hazel eyes, surprisingly smooth skin and high cheekbones, she had maintained the fierce determination that I remembered from a childhood that was punctuated with long mealtime sieges. I would be allowed to leave the table only when I surrendered and force-fed myself tapioca pudding, prunes and custard, or some other nauseating food.

Now she said 'Have a chat with Gwyneth.'

Gwyneth didn't look at me, but sighed and stretched her slim arms in the air so that the sleeves of her blue linen shirt fell in ripples down her arms.

Gwyneth, my mother's loyal friend, told me in a flat voice about the two occasions when a breast lump had turned out to be a harmless cyst. Then she stared at her narrow elegant feet in their navy high-heeled shoes.

'Yes, but mine's a hard lump', I said, and started to explain what I'd learned about the geology of body lumps.

Gwyneth shifted in her chair as I spoke, and looked away from me at a photograph of my mother in a rose silk coat standing next to my father after a school Speech Day, both of them surrounded by a group of school governors.

I added '... but my lump might turn out to be nothing at all.'

My mother returned. 'Gwyneth's told you, hasn't she', she said and the subject was closed. As far as my mother was concerned, my diagnosis was signed, sealed and delivered. I wasn't qualified to have the disease in the first place, so obviously the tests would reveal no positive results.

After my mother's edgy response, I was even more nervous about telling the children. My teenage daughter was still at school and my son and older daughter were still in their early twenties. I knew that I was a vital source of support to them, the strong mother that they could rely on to be consistent however much their current lives changed.

It would be foolish to worry them at this stage. It might be all for nothing. This waiting time was bad enough for me. Why inflict the worry on them? Why take away their faith in me unless it was absolutely necessary? If it did turn out to be cancer, I would tell them then. I myself was still trying to make sense of what cancer meant. It was all a jumble in my mind waiting to be processed. If I myself found it confusing, how could I possibly explain it to the children, let alone reassure them?

In reality, I was scared by the prospect of facing up to my children's pain – scared not just for them, but for me. I would find it painful to view their pain. My job was to protect them from pain, not be the cause of it.

We had moved house eight times since my son, my eldest child, was born, and the frequent moves over the years had made the children and me a tight unit. If I were diagnosed as a patient, the archetypal 'strong Welsh mother' role familiar to me since childhood might be lost. My children might feel that they had to protect me rather than the other way round. I just could not imagine such a reversal. The best thing was to carry on as normal and not let them know anything about what was going on. Most probably everything would turn out for the best and my results would clear me.

It was as if I was an accused mother awaiting a verdict of innocent or guilty. The results of the tests would be a verdict not only on my body but also on my vocation as a mother. Ever since I was a little girl growing up in Cymmer Afan, a tiny village in a South Wales valley, my ambition had always been the same. When I was six-years-old a school inspector asked me 'What do you want to be when you grow up?'

'A mother', I replied. Being a friend of my father's, the inspector duly reported this back to him. Thus it entered the annals of family mythology, the perpetual feedback of my career destiny as a mother.

Now I was facing a clash between my identity as a mother and my new identity as a patient. A mother is the warm centre of the household – a rock, selfless, and at the same time magical and intuitive so that she knows what is best for her children. This was the ideal I had picked up from my mother, my grandmother, my aunts and my friends' mothers when I was a little girl.

In 2001, Freeman and Brockmeier pointed out that 'One's personal identity, in so far as it is tied to the interpretive appraisal of one's personal past as it takes place in auto narrative, is inseparable from normative ideas of what a life is, or is supposed to be, if it is lived well.' My identity as a mother was inseparable from the Welsh 'mam', the frequently stereotyped domestic matriarch who is rooted in Welsh culture. Few of the mothers in Cymmer Afan had jobs, because there was little work for women in that small valley. For many mothers the chapel was their only non-domestic commitment. It was the home of the stirring sermon, the

Gymanfa Ganu (a festival of singing in four-part harmony) and the annual coach outing to the seaside at Barry or Aberavon. Although women played a vital part in the administration of the chapel, the learning and performing of the music and the Sunday-school teaching, it was men who ruled the roost. The minister was always male, as were the chapel elders, who sat in the 'Big Seat' that undulated around the elite area immediately below the pulpit.

In turn, the women claimed the domestic territory as their kingdom. My memories, romanticised by the passage of the years, were of women who scrubbed their front doorsteps, swept the streets outside their homes and motivated their children to perform well at school and in the chapel. They had a clear command of their territory and their goals. I grew up associating these mothers with a strong and powerful kind of femininity that emanated from strong and healthy female bodies. When I became a mother, I could feel that kind of femininity in my own body. Now I had the feeling that it would dissolve away if the medical tests failed to exonerate me.

CHAPTER 3

The verdict

The receptionist looked up at me and gave a professional smile. 'What time's your appointment?'

'It's for ten o'clock', Paul said. He took the appointment card from my hand and gave it to her, glancing sideways at me as he became aware of his habit of taking control in any medical setting.

The receptionist pointed back along the dimly lit corridor. 'You see that white door down there? Take a seat near it and you'll be called shortly.'

We walked back between the waiting patients and relatives who sat sidelined on black plastic chairs bordering the walls. At the far end of the corridor we came to the white door and sat down near it, facing an empty room with its door ajar. There was a sight chart on the wall opposite us, and we began to test each other to see how many of the lines we could read accurately: 'A E S I O.' When we reached the last line, we laughed as we each improvised the letters. I was relieved that we were carrying on in such a normal sort of way. The more normal our behaviour was, the more normal my results would be. Yet all the time my right leg was out of control, trembling and acting as the conduit for my fear that I might be tipped into the unknown world of cancer.

'Mrs Barnie?' A nurse emerged from behind the white door. A couple in their early seventies prised themselves out of their seats. The man was short and hunky and his wife was tiny and round with thick thighs that forced her to rock from side to side as she walked. He put his arm around her waist and guided her along the corridor.

'Take your time', said the nurse. Her lilting voice was familiar. It was Carys, a Breast Care nurse whom I'd met when accompanying Emma to a check-up. But she wasn't just a specialist breast cancer nurse – she was Welsh, a fellow exile and a locally renowned singer. Our shared Welshness and love of music was a good omen. She ushered the Barnies into the room behind the white door, leaving us to sit and wait for them to re-emerge.

There was a pink poster on the opposite wall giving information about Bosom Friends, 'the support group run by women with experience of breast cancer for women with breast cancer.' Emma was a member, as was Samira Khan, the woman whom I'd met at Rushwood Hospital when my lump was first tested.

'Anyone worried about breast cancer can call the Bosom Friends helpline', the poster announced. In that long gloomy corridor the poster was a sign that there were women out there thinking about me, women who knew what it was like to sit and wait endlessly for the consultant's verdict.

After a while Paul said 'It's ten thirty. Your appointment was for ten.'

'Yes. That woman, Mrs Barnie – she's been in there a long time. It must be bad news.'

I said this with difficulty, because my face had gone stiff and my right foot and knee were twitching up and down.

Selfish thoughts ran through my mind. 'If it's bad news for Mrs Barnie, does that make it more likely that it's good news for me? I don't want Mrs Barnie to have breast cancer. But if she has, it might mean that I haven't got it. I might be part of the good news in this clinic. How much bad news are they capable of giving? They wouldn't keep me waiting out here, agonising, hoping, not all this time, not if it were going to be bad news.'

At 10.45 the couple slowly emerged from the consulting room. Their faces were impassive, but Mr Barnie was now clinging to Mrs Barnie's arm as if he was afraid that she would drift away. Their fate was sealed. It was my turn now.

The consultant stood up, one large hand flicking back his brown curls. He shook our hands, smiled at me and pointed to the chair next to his desk. I sat down heavily. Paul sat on a chair a few feet away, while Carys was sitting in a far corner of the room in what seemed to be her appointed fail-safe position. The consultant made small talk for a few minutes, and I remembered our first meeting at Rushwood Hospital and my impressions of a sensitive, intelligent man. He was the sort of person in whom you could put your faith.

After a while the consultant, ignoring the other two, looked straight at me and began to talk about the tests. I watched his lips moving, monitoring what he said without listening. I was waiting, waiting for the words 'But it was not cancer.'

Then he looked into my eyes and said 'We have your results, and I'm sorry to tell you we have found cancer.'

I inhaled deeply. Along with sheer panic, an arrow of dislike flew out of me towards him. I'd put my faith in him, but now he had betrayed me.

But at the same time I knew that my reaction was irrational. I had put my trust in him, but it was a childish trust, counting on him not to tell me anything that would hurt me. Just as I had done with Gaia, my Internet muse. And just like Gaia, this was the real world.

Panic-stricken, I gazed out of the window opposite me at the flat blue sky. I stared and stared, riveted by it, and as I did so its flatness melted away and I became immersed in its infinite, absorbing depths. Words from Wordsworth's 'Tintern Abbey' came into my mind in a series of phrases and images that, beautiful though they were, had no cohesive meaning for me. They just added to my feeling that the moments of time were joining me, in my insignificance, not only to the abundance of nature but to all humanity:

> ... a sense sublime
> Of something far more deeply interfused,
> Whose dwelling is the light of setting suns,
> And the round ocean, and the living air,
> And the blue sky ...

I stared out of the window, motionless, aware that I was in a kind of a trance even as I was in it.

Eventually I tore my eyes away and tried to focus my attention back into the room. It was completely silent. The consultant was giving me time to take the news on board. He was unaware of the calming vision that had rescued me from the panic of the moment.

But it hadn't restored me to normality. Bemused and feeling dissociated from myself, I began to feel like a spectator. I was viewing the room's occupants as if I myself was not part of the scene. I was not that 'me' that was the object of the consultant's concern. In fact I was feeling sorry for 'she', the patient with the bad news, just as I was feeling sorry for the consultant. He had been given no choice but to give me bad news. My hostility to him vanished completely, and I admired his silent respect for the resonance of the occasion.

I couldn't really believe I had cancer. It was only a little lump. A cancerous lump, yes. But that didn't mean that my body had succumbed to the overwhelming concept of cancer.

I didn't feel important enough to have cancer. Cancer brings with it the special attentions of consultants, nurses, friends and family. It is a focal role, and I couldn't imagine myself in it long term, even though I'd spent the last couple of weeks reluctantly auditioning for it and even enjoying its drama from time to time.

The consultant started talking again. 'You'll need to start hormone treatment immediately and take it for five years. There are two possible surgical treatments and it's up to you which one you choose. Firstly, you can have an operation to remove the lump and the margins of tissue around it. You'll then need a six-week course of radiotherapy.'

He paused, 'The other option is to have a mastectomy, to remove the entire breast tissue.'

'Yes, yes. That's what I want. Get rid of the breast altogether.'

At last I'd managed to speak. Until then everything had been too complicated, but now I could physically feel the sense of this simple option, a clean sweep of the knife that both avenged my breast for letting me down and sliced out the deadly cancer at the same time.

The consultant said 'Either way, you will have an operation in about two weeks, a lumpectomy of the right breast or a mastectomy. And either way, you might need chemotherapy afterwards. During the operation we'll remove the lymph nodes from under your arm. If you have a mastectomy you may not need radiotherapy after the operation. On the other hand, a mastectomy is a major procedure and research shows that a lumpectomy followed by radiotherapy gives every bit as good a prognosis in cases like yours.'

'No, I'd rather have a mastectomy.'

'Well, you don't need to decide now – you can think about it for a few days. Now then, would you like to go with Carys and make an appointment to come and see her later this week? You'll be able to talk things over with her.'

'No thanks. I'll be all right.'

The energy had drained out of me and I couldn't imagine returning so soon to that hospital, the fount of my bad news.

The consultant and Carys exchanged glances. I had misread the consultant's politeness. I could see that it was not only usual but mandatory to return for a follow-up session with Carys.

'Hm, I think you'd find it helpful.'

'Sure I will. Yes, thank you.'

The consultant shook my hand and said he'd see me in a couple of weeks. 'Don't worry. It looks as though you have a good prognosis' he repeated, and he gave me a small smile.

I believed him, even as I remembered his confidence at our first meeting that my lump was unlikely to be a tumour.

Carys beckoned us into an anteroom. We sat down in front of a small pine table that had a box half full of pink paper tissues as a centrepiece, like an offering on an altar. I slumped into the chair.

Carys, my handmaiden, hovered beside me. 'Are you all right?'

I nodded as a cool trail of wetness wended its way down my hot cheeks – yet more tears for the paper tissues.

'I'll go and get you some water.' Carys, practised in the ritual, left the room. Paul put his arm around me.

'You're doing really well.'

I blinked the tears away. 'I don't know why those tears came. Maybe it was the sight of that box of tissues, like a cue – "Hey there, it's crying time." But I'm OK now.'

It wasn't until we stepped outside the hospital that it hit me. The sun was still shining in a pure blue sky, just as it had been nearly two hours ago. But now I was a different person. I was now a patient. It was official. I felt no sicker than before my consultation. In fact, I felt perfectly healthy. The only change was that the consultant had delivered his verdict. He had the power to turn me into an authenticated patient. I now had a medical label. I was a 'cancer patient', one of the many who passed through the hospital every year. Not only would I have to think of myself as a patient – I'd also have to get used to others seeing me as a patient as well.

On the way home from the hospital it crossed my mind that I could still keep the whole thing secret. Then I could carry on being the same person and I wouldn't have to put up with others looking at me in a different light, as a patient. I just wanted to stay the same person, to come out at the end of whatever was in store for me and be the same person as when it all started. This would be much easier if others had never known about my illness anyway.

A friend had hidden her illness and told others only when her chemotherapy was over. And I'd read a newspaper article about a beauty editor on a glossy magazine who had worked throughout her chemotherapy and radiotherapy and confided in friends and family only weeks before her death. Was that what a good patient did? Maybe my idea of hiding my diagnosis wasn't just selfish. Maybe the good patient soldiers on, keeping it all secret and sheltering those close to her from the realities of her illness.

But looking at it realistically, I knew I didn't have the type of personality that could keep up that kind of facade – especially with all the energy and discretion that it needed. Yet I couldn't let the idea go.

On the way home from hospital, my mind played with the relative merits of disclosing and not disclosing my illness:

Yes, I will keep my diagnosis a secret.

- *It will help me stay the same person and enable me to carry on as though nothing has happened.*
- *It will protect the children so that they don't have to worry about me.*
- *In the eyes of my family (Paul excepted), friends and colleagues, I will still be a healthy woman, the same person they have always known.*
- *I won't have to worry about telling others about my illness only to find that I have embarrassed them.*
- *I'm more likely to keep my job if I return to work and carry on as normally as possible.*

Yes, I will tell everyone about my illness.

- *I won't have to hide my feelings or what is going on in my body and my life – less hassle, less stress.*
- *I'll enjoy the support of my family and friends and be closer to them.*
- *I'll be able to share symptoms with my fellow patients and bond with them.*
- *If I don't tell everyone about my diagnosis, they might find out anyway and be hurt that I hadn't confided in them.*
- *I won't have to keep up appearances by returning to work when my instincts are telling me to take time off until the treatment is over.*

Looking back, I can see that by weighing up the two options I was working out what sickness meant to me at that point. Non-disclosure seemed to offer the chance to avoid being seen as abnormal by others and to leave things as they were. That way my relationships with others would remain unchanged, my life would stay the same and, most important of all, my sense of self as an independent and efficiently functioning person would not be disrupted. I could be the same mother, friend and worker, and my sickness would be just a small addendum in my life, one that need not impinge on my real life and my real self, and that would spare me two out of the three elements of the crisis that Brody (2003) has described:

> To be sick is to participate in a disruption of an integrated hierarchy of natural systems, including one's biological subsystems, oneself as a discrete psychological entity and the social and cultural systems of which one is a member.

Biological disruption was unavoidable, but might I be able to sidestep some of the psychological and social consequences of my diagnosis? No, enticing as it was, I realised the hopelessness of opting for the tensions, the pretences and the complications of non-disclosure. Yet my mind was reluctant to dismiss the notion altogether. Maybe I could mix and match – tell some people and not others. No, that would be madness. No, much as I'd like to keep my illness completely secret, I'd have to take the most straightforward option and just tell everyone who might be interested.

Soon after I got home I rang my mother.

'It's cancer.'

'Are they sure?'

'Yes, they are, I'm afraid.'

In the silence I could feel our relationship changing. My mother, although strong and energetic, had two artificial hips and was unsteady on her feet. I had always begun our phone calls by asking how she was, the understanding being that she was the vulnerable one. Now, although she was 82, her life expectancy might be greater than mine – after all, her problems were mechanical rather than organic.

I tried to cheer her up.

'I'm seeing Carys, the Breast Care nurse, on Friday for a counselling session.'

'Good ... a counselling session.'

My mother sounded relieved. It sounded so mysterious and yet positive, as if something magical would happen.

After I had put the phone down, I was conscious of a frantic energy in my mind and body, arising from the kind of hysteria that a crisis induces. Whatever its source, I might just as well make the most of it while it lasted.

I rang friend after friend, perpetuating what had become a ritual. It was only a year since my friend Emma had done the same thing and rung mostly the same friends, to give mostly the same message. The year before that another friend had been diagnosed with cancer. Although each of us friends might fixate on our own individual health indicators out of all those that the media tossed around – gym-honed fitness, safe sex, religious affiliation, eating spinach, drinking cider vinegar, saying no to drugs, or even just comparative youth – there was no getting away from the fact that illness was still for the most part random and unpredictable.

The responses to my calls were a warm blanket of sympathy except for one friend, Charlie, who said 'You're the third with cancer. I visited Richard Ellis in hospital last Monday and I doubt he's got long. And then John Salt, do you know him? Brilliant snooker player. He's got a brain tumour.'

How depressing. Instead of relating my bad news uniquely to me, Charlie had assigned me to a team of players whom I had never met. I was now one of 'them', those cancer victims – me, Richard, Johnny and unknown others. Sympathy suddenly seemed like a double-edged sword, capable of making me feel loved or rejected with the implication that 'You're sick and I'm not.'

I had the same feeling that I had experienced when I first met my consultant and he fitted my story into a format that suited him and the hospital system, based on his medical knowledge and experience, his role in the medical hierarchy, the administrative systems and the desire to avoid wasting time. Even as I had recognised the need for scientific rigour, efficiency and financial economy, I had felt as if my story was out of my control. Now Charlie was fitting my story into another template, probably one of many that I was going to come across.

No wonder that Emma had once confided in me that everyone has their own concept of cancer and 'Sometimes you can feel the presence of their idea of cancer like a kind of third person in the room.'

Now, post-diagnosis, I had no choice but to tell the children. I told them one by one but in such an upbeat way that they were left completely confused. They were unsure whether the diagnosis was anything to worry about or not, although they only told me about their confusion months later when I was less jittery. At the time, I was so uneasy about using the word 'cancer' and its associations of death in relation to myself, and having it intrude into my relationship with the children, that I minimised its significance.

The gist of what I said was 'I've got breast cancer but it's not serious and I'll soon be better.'

I wanted to separate my disease from all the associations with the word 'cancer' that the children would almost certainly have already absorbed. In her book *Teratologies*, Jackie Stacey describes my fear of the word 'cancer' and the stigma that it carries as 'a symptom of the pervasive forms of cultural anxiety.' It was a learned fear, something that I had absorbed from many sources, including the media, friends and family. And now this symptom of cultural anxiety was meeting another. My fear of illness was meeting my fear of failing to live up to the ideal that I had carried with me from Cymmer Afan, my childhood village – the ideal of the dedicated and impregnable mother.

Ceri, my younger daughter, was with me when my friend, Emma, came round one evening bearing a huge bunch of pink roses and a card with the inscription 'With love from one survivor to another.' This message was my first glimpse into something that helped me through my treatment, namely the female bonding that can arise from shared suffering, especially between close friends. Yes, like Emma I was going to fight this disease and survive it. We would face it together.

But then I looked at the inscription again. The word 'survivor' implied that I was facing danger. It also implied that the outcome of my illness was self-determined. After all, to be a survivor means to do something active to ensure that one survives. Yet I wasn't sure what I personally could do against my cancer to ensure my survival. I was familiar with the idea of 'fighting it', but what was I supposed to do other than comply with my treatment? I had read about the importance of 'positive thinking' but had also noticed, to my disappointment, that there was little scientific evidence to link it with any cancer outcome. Just as I had been torn between hiding my cancer or making it public, so I was now torn between my longing to believe in self-empowering claims to cure it and my scepticism about claims that weren't scientifically proven.

Diagnosis had always seemed to me to be a final and clear-cut event, an end to speculation and a clear path forward. Now it was turning out that there were many optional paths that followed it, and many choices to be made. What should I make of my diagnosis? What stance should I take in relation to my illness? Which treatment should I choose? So many options when the only thing I was sure about was that I wanted to get this illness over with and then get on with my life once more.

I began to worry in case Ceri saw the card with its disturbing description of me as a 'survivor.' I took the pink roses into the kitchen to put them in a vase, and hid the card under the clutter in one of the kitchen drawers. As I did so there came a faint memory of the time when my mother had enlisted Gwyneth's help in insisting that my lump was a benign cyst. Like her, I was tidying the threat away.

CHAPTER 4

Time out

The morning after my diagnosis we visited a local stately home. An outing in the country, Paul and I had agreed, would take my mind off the shock of my diagnosis for a few hours and then I would be able to make a cool-headed choice between my treatment options – lumpectomy or mastectomy. It seemed a rational enough plan at the time, but as it turned out, it was misguided.

At the end of a leafy drive, Middleton Hall came into view, a gleaming white mansion house with tall, sixteenth-century windows. To our left there was a sudden rumbling noise and out of the greenery emerged a white-haired man in his late seventies. His blue denim shirt and black jeans were slightly dusty, and he was pushing a wheelbarrow piled high with planks of wood.

He stopped when he saw us. 'Hello there. Welcome to the estate. Have you come to take a look around?'

He didn't wait for an answer.

'My name is Nicholas. I'd be happy to be your guide and show you what's going on round here if you like.'

He spoke with the plummy accent of an English landowner, one who had seemingly fallen on hard times.

'Yes please, we'd like that', I said.

After the previous day's encounter with the consultant, I was still feeling intimidated by anyone associated with authority. Paul gave me a straight-lipped smile, eyebrows lifted. We'd been hoping to wander around in a casual sort of way and just enjoy the ambience of the place.

Nicholas parked his wheelbarrow under a tree and strolled along with us.

I looked up at him. I am five feet eight inches tall but he towered nearly half a foot above me.

'I suppose you're the owner of the estate?'

'No, I used to be a barrister. Now I'm happy just to be one of the workforce.'

He pointed to his left towards a barn. A group of elderly men were measuring up and sawing wood.

'Those are my workmates. We're all volunteers trying to get this place shipshape again. It's going to take a few more years. I just hope I'll still be around to see the final results.'

It was difficult to concentrate on what he was saying. It sounded extraneous compared with the obsessive thoughts that were spinning around in my head. Nicholas was the only stranger I'd met since my diagnosis the previous day. He knew nothing about my cancer. As far as I could tell, he thought that I was a normal person, yet I was feeling completely disoriented by my new cancer-positive state. If I had broken my arm he would have seen the plaster and known I was injured, but instead I looked completely normal. He knew nothing and saw only this quiet woman, the subdued but healthy-seeming me. I felt like a fraud – as if I were trying to pass as a healthy woman when in fact I wasn't. I wanted to tell Nicholas the reality because I wanted a reaction – any reaction – from him. But giving him inappropriately personal news about my illness would only embarrass him.

It had been a mistake to venture out so soon after my diagnosis. It would have been wiser to stay at home for a while and practise being a patient. At the hospital it was easy to be a patient because other people fed me my role. At home I was easing myself into the patient role, helped by friends and family. Here I was on alien ground with no idea of how to be a patient in the outside world. It was tempting to make an excuse to Nicholas and put an end to this guided tour – but then again it was probably best just to carry on politely playing the role of the interested tourist and see this encounter through to its end.

As Nicholas led us up the wide stone steps of the building, his wiry frame striding forward above us, I became aware of him as a survivor. He was someone who was here, living in the world, when many of his friends were already dead.

People's lives are usually measured in terms of their quality rather than their length. Not one of the Brontë sisters reached the age of 40, cellist Jacqueline du Pré was only 42 when she died of multiple sclerosis, Dinah Washington, the blues and gospel singer, was 39, and the rock star Janis Joplin was just 27. Yet their respective books and music have ensured them a kind of timelessness.

So yes, an individual's life is measured by more than its longevity, but now for the first time in my life I admired someone – even envied them – for just carrying on living. I wanted to be like Nicholas. I wanted to live a long time. Hierarchies exist everywhere where humans gather. Why had I never realised before that there is a hierarchy of lifespan?

Living a long time, however dysfunctional or painful the experience, suddenly seemed to me to be an achievement in itself – the achievement of still living, still learning, still being there for and with family and friends long after other less fortunate contemporaries had passed away.

There was a map in my mind that showed the trail of my life ending when I was in my eighties. I had expected to live at least as long as my mother and grandmothers, perhaps even longer. I could see now that this was a dream, not a reality. The 'me' whom I had thought about and hoped to become in future years might never happen. I might never be a grandmother, never spend more time composing music for cello and piano, never visit the remote countries that I had listed hopefully in my diary. All the plans that had formed in my mind with the constancy of facts might already be pure fiction as far as my body was concerned.

The only 'facts' related to what had happened in my life already and what was happening now. The path I had been following was an imaginary one, and now what the future held was uncertain, so that I was filled with misty fears. 'Somehow the stories we have in place never fit the reality', wrote Frank in *The Wounded Storyteller*, 'and sometimes this disjunction can be worse than having no story at all.'

'This is the Great Hall.' Nicholas extended his arm and my attention flicked back to the present.

'This used to be home to Sir Francis Willoughby, naturalist and founder of the Royal Society. He was only 37 when he died in 1672.'

Only 37 and he had already achieved so much. But what about me? I could be dead in a couple of years and what had I achieved? In common with many women, I was fairly accomplished on the personal front – bringing up three children, caring for them, entertaining them, motivating them, working full- or part-time hours as fitted in with the family, and helping Paul in his career. But when it came to the public domain, my lecturing, writing and sporadic music gigs counted for little. I was going to die and disappear into a void. Life would carry on as usual without me. My life had been local and private and would pass with only local and private acknowledgement. It was as if I had played at a concert and then found out that only the front row of the audience could hear me.

But these feelings of panic and regret quickly receded. Why was I so concerned? Suddenly my real values in life seemed to have gone out of the window and I was desperate to be remembered by strangers. It was as if I were a ghost, and the real me, grounded in my everyday life, had vanished in the aristocratic setting of Middleton Hall.

'His distinguished colleague, John Ray, also lived here for a time', Nicholas was saying.

'You might have heard of him because he devised the system of classifying flora and fauna that is still used today.'

'How old was he when he died?' I asked.

'He was 78 and still working as a theological scientific writer.'

Seventy-eight ... over twice as old as Sir Francis when he died.

When I got home I couldn't stop brooding over the duration of people's lives. When Sir Francis died in 1672, John Ray was 45 and his work and life story carried on for a further 33 years. Two men with different life histories. No women – although Nicholas had referred to their wives, they didn't really figure in his story, and the socio-political implications of their omission were of no interest to me. I was too obsessed with their husbands' contrasting life spans. Pre-diagnosis, it would never have occurred to me to notice whether one historic figure lived longer than another. Now I was obsessed with the statistics and I too wanted lots of time, just like John Ray. I began to think about all the time that I had already wasted in my life – time when I had felt depressed and had just done the bare minimum to get through every-day life, or even just happily wasted time doing nothing. What was I doing frittering away my time as if I had so much of it to spare?

Time is complex and is more than its measurements. It can pass slowly or quickly. This wake-up call would mean that I would never squander time again. From now on time and life would always be precious to me and I would always strive to make the best of them.

It was then that the idea struck me. From now on I would make the best of things, and take control of things, by learning how to be a good patient. I would try to lead as good a life as is compatible with being a patient. That way I would have a purpose that would help me to rise above setbacks. That way I wouldn't get bogged down in my own petty worries as I had today. And, most important of all, that way I would deserve to stay my old unchanged self, albeit with a new and more realistic take on life.

It felt like a pact with fate. I would offer up my life as a good patient as a lucky charm so that I could remain my old familiar self and return to my old familiar life at the end of my treatment.

CHAPTER 5

Decisions

Decisions are snake-like things. My mind kept coiling ever farther into itself as I tried to make a decision that would give me the very best chance of living as long as I possibly could. My choice was between two different treatment plans – mastectomy alone or lumpectomy followed by radiotherapy.

In either case, I might also need a course of chemotherapy, depending on my results after surgery. It was up to me to weigh up the two alternatives and decide which one gave me the better chance of surviving my cancer.

Patient choice. Big deal. I was going along with the system because this choice business had obviously evolved over time and maybe there was more to it than I knew about. Nevertheless, the very fact that I had been given a choice niggled me. Why was I, a mere patient, being asked to choose between two different treatment plans? I knew little about the complexities involved, so I could only make an uneducated guess at the right choice. The doctors know the science, the statistics and the latest expert thinking on the subject. They are practitioners in the world of cancer treatment and research. Surely it is their job as experts – these oncologists, surgeons, pathologists and whoever – to pool their knowledge, weigh up the complex pros and cons and come to a decision. For some reason they weren't going to do this. Well, if they weren't going to do it, I would have to feel my way to a decision as best I could, by myself.

Two days previously, in the Wednesday clinic, my consultant had presented the equivalence of the two treatment plans in a positive and absolute way. Both were so good that it didn't really matter which one I chose. I wanted to go along with this, wanted to believe it, but I had the feeling that I was only being given the choice because medical research had failed to establish which was the better treatment for patients in my situation – mastectomy on the one hand, or lumpectomy followed by radiotherapy on the other. This lack of fine discrimination could only be due to insufficient current information.

I was used to consumer reports on technological systems such as vacuum cleaners or computers, reports that ranked their results in order of efficacy. There was rarely a dead heat even though they were comparing like with like – washing machine with washing machine, toaster with toaster.

The choice that I was being offered was not between like and like but between two completely different treatment regimes. It seemed to me that it was improbable that they were equally effective.

It was reassuring in many ways that the medics were sharing the complexity of medical treatment and decisions with their patients. They were recognising the need to step down from their professionally detached role, to engage with their patients and to encourage them to take responsibility for what happens to their bodies.

Alas, I had the feeling that the choice my consultant had offered me might turn out to be a poisoned chalice, in that whatever decision I made, I might eventually start to question it or even regret it.

What is more, the process itself seemed to me to be imperfect – too little information and too little time. I had been given two days in which to make up my mind, with no input of information apart from what the consultant had told me in my emotionally fraught, 'Sorry but you've got breast cancer' consultation, and apart from a booklet about breast cancer that included three sentences explaining mastectomy and three explaining lumpectomy.

All in all, I felt overwhelmed by the responsibility of the choice that I had to make, and I began to long for that old discredited paternalism in which the all-powerful consultant spelled out to the blindly trusting patient exactly what treatment was going to be given. The doctor's Foucaldian clinical gaze, born of the ability to see through to the truth, had been replaced in my case by the patient's baffled stare. Yes, ideally I wanted to make the decision for myself, and I welcomed the way in which my autonomy was being respected. But at the same time I wanted a lot of input from the experts. They were the ones who, unlike me, had a scientific training, were emotionally unengaged in my illness and had the 'group rationality', described by Schneider in *The Practice of Autonomy*, that comes from being part of a scientific culture and its norms, based on academic literature and refined practice.

Schneider, an expert on patient autonomy, found that what most people want from their doctor is competence and kindness. Most doctors are competent and kind, but what Schneider had in mind was the kind of fused combination that responds with acuity to patients across the range of their needs. There are patients like me who need to share the decision-making process, and there are those who welcome complete control over the making of vital decisions. Some patients are too tired or too depressed to want to take part in the decision making, or do not wish to for other reasons. In each of these cases, the process that leads to the decision will vary according to the individualistic needs and intentions of the patient, but in each case the patient has made an autonomous choice.

Of course such a complex process cannot be one-sided. It was no use my wishing that my consultant and I had engaged in this intricate kind of power-sharing exercise, because I had given him no opportunity to initiate one. The patient should surely take some responsibility, too, and not just leave everything to the doctor so that he has to guess the patient's needs. I should have asked some questions and shown that I was open to information. Instead I had been too emotional and I had neurotically fixated on a mastectomy, irrespective of other factors. Now I would have to make the best of it and muddle through the decision making as best I could.

On Friday, the day of my hospital appointment, I was still mulling over my choice of treatment as I loaded the breakfast dishes into the dishwasher. Would it be better to amputate the whole faulty breast or to excise only the unwanted tumour and its surrounding flesh, leaving the rest of the breast intact? That very afternoon, at four o'clock, I would have to give my final decision to Carys, the specialist Breast Care nurse, so that the arrangements for the appropriate operation could go ahead.

It was then that I remembered the other decision, the secret one that I had taken after my visit to Middleton Hall the previous day – the decision to be a good patient. Immediately my view of my dilemma started to change. It was no longer depressing and purely personal – it had become part of a project.

I would approach the choice as a good patient would. I would look at the challenge from all angles and make an objective, logical decision based on my research.

I jotted down a brief list of the factors that I should take into consideration when weighing up the issues:

- *factor 1* – what the consultant had told me
- *factor 2* – the information I gained from Gaia
- *factor 3* – advice and information from Paul, friends and family.

Concerning factor 1, what *had* the consultant told me? The important facts as I had seen them were seared in my memory, but I wasn't sure that they included many medical details relevant to the decision. The only fact I was sure of, and it was an important one, was that the consultant had said that, in cases like mine, statistics showed that a lumpectomy followed by radiotherapy led to the same life expectancy as a mastectomy.

I also had a feeling that he had said that a lumpectomy was more breast conserving and more femininity conserving, as it would leave my body more or less intact. So factor 1 was straightforward – go for a lumpectomy.

Factor 2 was equally conclusive. Gaia came up with a range of reputable sites that cited research proving that, for suitable cases, each regime resulted in the same life expectancy. Given this fact, lumpectomy was again the treatment of choice.

Factor 3 moved into a grey area. As a by-product of my investigations into factor 2, I had found some research which claims that most patients actually prefer to be given a choice of treatment. This surprised me. None of the friends who had phoned, emailed or visited me since my diagnosis had expected me to welcome being given a choice. A couple of women friends who had themselves experienced serious illness even questioned whether the consultant had given me the complete picture. I listened to them carefully.

It turned out that I had failed to act as a streetwise patient and ask a male, married consultant the killer question with regard to being given a choice: 'What would you advise your wife to do in my situation, doctor?'

It had not occurred to me to ask it, but now I wished that I had, because I could see the point of it. I began to worry that the consultant had been too influenced by the femininity and conservationist angle of lumpectomy, and included it in his comparison of the efficacy of the two treatments instead of just regarding it as a welcome extra. He might have thought that it was more important to me than it actually was. If I had asked the killer question, would it have affected the consultant's thoughts for a moment?

Women are used to being asked all kinds of personal questions by male doctors whose own personal lives are hidden, and all the cancer specialists at Parkside Hospital were male at that time. It takes some bravado to ask such a personal question of a doctor, even if it is only one that implicitly casts the patient in the cosy familial role of 'wife.' I admired those women who had dared to ask it. It is a question which implies that the doctor has some information that he is holding back. His own wife would benefit from his knowledge and convictions, but he gives his patients a spurious choice in order to comply with unknown pressures. By asking the question, the patient is trying to identify herself with his wife in order to find out the real truth.

The fact that some consultants then respond by giving their personal opinions only confirms the ambiguity of this scenario. What does it mean? Is the consultant now giving an opinion that is based on the experience that he has amassed, the theory that he has studied, or what?

Because I had already learned that the doctor, the fount of medical knowledge, had the power to withhold as well as to disclose information, I shared the uncertainties that led to the question, even though I hadn't thought of asking it.

All had seemed straightforward when I examined factors 1 and 2, but now everything was getting complicated and I had strayed into areas that might be important or might be totally irrelevant. I might be getting bogged down in obscure issues, and I was not getting anywhere with my decision. I felt isolated in a new, 'uncool' world of illness – a world that was shunned by fit, healthy people.

In no time at all I found myself downstairs sitting at the piano, my flight response to stress activated before I knew it. I played a few minor chords in the bass with my left hand and sang 'Mast–ec–tomy, lump–ec–tomy; lump–ec–tomy, mast–ec–tomy', each word lingering over a crotchet, a dotted crotchet, a quaver and another crotchet. I jazzed up the rhythm and hummed along to it. Maybe someone should write *Cancer: the Musical*. It was dramatic enough, with all of its difficult decisions, and it was certainly universal enough. There could be few people who didn't know someone with cancer.

Well, then again, maybe not. Who would write a drama about illness? Well, Dennis Potter, the playwright, for one. I thought of his hero in *The Singing Detective*, who suffers from acute psoriasis and side-effects associated with his treatment. In hospital, he deliriously tries to figure out who he is and how he got into that terrible situation. Watching him before I was ill, I hadn't realised that I was watching in innocence, that I was not grasping the depths of the invalid role, the helplessness, the fears and the desperate hopes involved in being a patient. With my new experience of illness, I realised that even now I had only been given a glimpse into the suffering caused by his illness, and that I was learning the limits of empathy.

Other dramas that portrayed illness or disability came into my mind. *My Left Foot*, the film of the true story of Christy Brown, who was part of a large Irish family and was paralysed from birth as a result of cerebral palsy. Helped by his mother, Brown's courage and determination enable him to learn to read, and to write with the one limb that he can control – his left foot. He grows up to become a well-known author, painter and fundraiser.

Yes, I'd forgotten. Illness can be portrayed live on stage and screen, acted out by boisterous teams of people and shown to be part of normal life.

I returned to my desk and my dilemma feeling more resolute. Once more my thoughts returned to factor 3 in a bid to get this decision over with once and for all. Neither friends nor family had shown any desire to influence my actual choice of treatment, least of all Paul. He was a general practitioner – a specialist in primary care, not in the latest refinements of hospital-based cancer treatment – and he preferred the decision to rest with me and my consultant.

Yet most of my friends took it for granted that my final choice about treatment would be Paul's decision.

'Paul must know all about it', they said. 'What has Paul told you to do?'

They saw him as the expert on my disease – a doctor trained in medical information – and me as the disease's uncomprehending victim, and I resented being typecast, despite the fact that however much I consulted Gaia, I often viewed myself in this way.

Now it was time to return yet again to Gaia, this time to find out more about what a mastectomy involved. I knew little about it but there were many sites – those of charities, the NHS and even the BBC – providing information for laypeople like me.

Public websites like these represented the main category of mastectomy-related sites, but there were two other significant ones, both commercial. I discovered that the mastectomy industry was big, especially in America. Companies with names like 'Sweet Dreams' or 'Bare Necessities' were selling post-mastectomy bras and other lingerie, and cosmetic surgeons were selling post-mastectomy reconstructions.

Some of the cosmetic surgery sites had 'before' and 'after' pictures of women who had had mastectomies. Looking at them I began to see them through the prism of cosmetic surgery. The scarred, mastectomised side could be returned to 'normal' by the doctors. It could be built up and matched to the other side, and the woman would appear to have exactly the same body as she had before her operation. It seemed that post mastectomy a great deal of energy must be directed towards covering up the signs of disease and treatment in order to retain one's femininity. It looked like the same kind of pressure that I had newly detected in the women's magazines, but at the same time it was reassuring that the option was there to 'normalise' my body if I opted for mastectomy.

Then I came across a website that had a photograph of the writer, Deena Metzger. It showed her naked from the hips up, standing against the clouds and sky. Her arms were stretched straight out and she was looking up towards the sky. Across the scar on the right side of her chest there was a tattoo of a tree branch. The photograph had been taken by the photographer Hella Hammid in 1978, and it portrayed her as healthy, vital and heroic. I looked for more images like this, since this was now the twenty-first century and such images must be commonplace. However, this was the only image of a mastectomy that I came across where it was presented as a valid choice and complete in itself, emphasising the woman's option to choose reconstruction or not.

This image was inspirational. Mastectomy was not the masochistic, body-avenging choice that I had envisaged in my first panic after diagnosis. It could be a statement about dignity and the nature of femininity. What is more, it would give the reassurance that I still hankered after – the reassurance of feeling that all my suspect flesh had been eradicated.

But it was no good. I was too scared to have a mastectomy, too unsure of how I would react to a body that would be so altered. I had always avoided knowing the details of how my body worked. Doctors regard the body as an ultra-efficient machine, but I had the superstitious belief that it was a mystical thing, and I tried to disregard the bones and organs that lay beneath its skin and flesh. Post mastectomy it would be disturbing to touch the surgically flattened area, to feel skin newly touching bone that had once lain hidden deep. A lumpectomy would remove only a wide rim of tissue surrounding the lump, leaving the hidden mystery beneath intact.

On the other hand, just over a year ago Emma had discovered a breast lump and had been operated on just five days after being seen by the consultant. She had been given no choice about her mastectomy, and she had nobly shrugged it off in public, joking and generally carrying on as normal. She had successfully completed the rest of her treatment and now she was an upbeat role model for me. Why not follow her example as best I could? Especially since if I did, I wouldn't have to endure weeks of radiotherapy at a later date.

No, I couldn't go through with it. My emotions were winning, and luckily I had a choice – I could indulge my fear of a mastectomy.

What is more, thinking back to Wednesday's consultation, it now seemed to me that the consultant, with all his experience and knowledge, had been encouraging me to consider a lumpectomy. With all his expertise and experience, he probably had some insight into my mind as well as my body – insight that led him to know that lumpectomy was the best choice for me.

Everything had already changed so much – my everyday life with its hospital visits and my long consultations with Gaia, my relationships with my friends and family, and even my relationship with my future now that it had been exposed as a cosy dream. Best to minimise any other changes.

It was as if I was having to choose between two new incarnations of myself – the one with a mastectomy and the one with a lumpectomy. I would be someone different according to which choice I made. It was frightening, and I decided to go for the less radical option, the one that I hoped would impose minimal changes on my mind and my body and leave me as my same self, the same mother of my children, the same woman, body and soul.

So in the end it was my emotional responses that swung my decision, but only after numerous activities, including recapping on what I could remember of the consultant's words, guessing what he was thinking, listening to friends and family, surfing through all the data, and losing myself in a morass of unfathomable detail. My attempt to act the part of the good patient and sort out the relevant information before coming to a logical decision had coalesced and dive-bombed into an intuitive choice – lumpectomy. I just hoped that it wasn't a decision which I would regret later when it was too late.

CHAPTER 6

Revelations

I was back in that same narrow hospital corridor where I'd waited to hear the news about my diagnosis. This time I had an appointment with Carys, my nurse specialist. Although it seemed like a lifetime later, it was just two days since my last visit, and in that time I had finally made up my mind about my choice of treatment. Far from making a rational decision after weighing up all the pros and cons, it had been a messy, emotional business, and in the end I had abandoned information and logic and gone for a verdict based on my uncertainties and a kind of sixth sense. I had opted for a 'lump–ec–tomy.'

Seated on a hard plastic chair next to an elderly, sleeping woman, I looked about me, and my perspective on my decision began to grow softer. Amid the harsh straight lines of the corridor and its plain, pale walls, I began to see myself as yet another vulnerable, complex patient, dusted with the dark richness of life outside the hospital. After making a complex decision in critical circumstances, I now had time to ponder the process, and I realised that I had done more than passively rely on my sixth sense. During the two days since my last visit I had acquired at least some of the information that was necessary in order to weigh up my decision rationally. Gaia had given me some medical facts and explanations. I had remembered odd pieces of information that the consultant had given me, and I had talked to Emma and other friends who had suffered serious illness. All the 'logic' resulting from this information had gone into my subconscious and contributed to my 'intuitive' decision of the heart. And what did I mean by my sixth sense other than a decision that took into account my own experience and values? They all served to complement the 'facts.' They were all important factors. My decision was based on sundry factors, but it was not the completely irrational one that I had originally thought it was.

Deciding on my choice of treatment had proved to be anything but simple, and in many ways I was more confused at the end of the process than at the beginning. Yet it had not been a completely negative experience. It had prodded me into learning new information not only about my treatment but also about myself. It had given me more insight into the staff and the institution that had given me the choice, and this knowledge would help me when it came to understanding and negotiating my way through the course of my treatment. Although slightly disappointed with the way in which I'd handled it, I remained optimistic. The dilemma itself might have made a better patient out of me.

The decision about my treatment was a public one that I was about to divulge to the medical staff, but there was also the second, secret decision to think about – the one that had first come to mind during my visit to Middleton Hall the previous day. There I had decided to be a good patient and to lead as good a life as possible that was compatible with being a patient. First, this decision was a pact with fate, a lucky charm – if I lived as a good patient then I would deserve to remain unchanged, to be the same person at the end of my treatment as at the beginning. Secondly, it reflected the curiosity that edged my fear. It was the kind of curiosity that comes with a new job. What would it be like to be a patient? What would I need to do to be successful at it? What were the criteria and the qualities needed? Who would I have to be? Lastly, my secret decision was a strategy for survival. It was an optimistic aim to bolster me through the unknown events that were in store for me and to give meaning to my time in limbo. That way my identity would not just depend on the medical professionals who I would meet in the clinic and on the hospital ward, but also on the examples of other patients – inside and outside the hospital, past and present – and on their ways of living. This was my private decision, the one I would keep to myself.

There was a brief hush. Dark curls rippling, my consultant was loping along the corridor to his consulting room at the far end. I was ready to greet him as he passed by, but he kept his eyes fixed firmly ahead, avoiding any possibility of acknowledging the ill people sitting to the side of him. In that moment I saw not an arrogant consultant but a man under pressure. He was the hunted quarry and all we patients lining the walls, old and young and in different stages of illness, were the hunters – yearning, needy and hoping to get what we had come for.

Outside the clinic, the course of the consultant's working day was a mystery to us, and we could only guess at the hours spent operating, examining X-rays, scans and pathology results, doing ward rounds and liaising with other staff. But here in the clinic, for a brief time, he was ours. In this locality he was face to face with our expectations, and it was not easy for him. We patients all had different needs and different expectations, and he had to identify these and respond to each of them as best he could while working under time constraints. I was looking through the doctor's eyes, like the hijacked victim who comes to identify with their captor, except that the consultant was not my captor but my rescuer.

I thought of Anna, a friend who had been diagnosed with breast cancer 13 years previously, who had assured me that things had improved since she was diagnosed. She had been given just two bare facts with no explanation: 'You've got cancer and you'll be starting chemotherapy.'

She was terrified because everyone she knew who had been given chemotherapy had died, including her mother. When she asked a question about her treatment, her consultant had said 'You don't want to go into all that.' The implication was that the doctor owned the information about her cancer, and it would do her no good to hear it.

Things were different now, but the changes didn't make the doctors' jobs any easier, because they now faced the challenge of giving explanations tailored to the needs of the individual patient.

I began to see why some doctors would feel obliged to answer that popular question that so many women patients asked 'What would you advise your wife to do, doctor?' Trained to answer patients' questions, they would be tempted to respond out of sympathy with the bewildered patient, despite the fact that any response other than an evasive one would by its very nature be personal and therefore unprofessional. Doctors, thankfully, are vulnerable, too.

Despite this fleeting feeling of empathy with my consultant, I felt disappointed that he had arranged for me to give my decision to the specialist nurse and not to him. Was it because in the hierarchical organisation of the hospital, information that the consultant chooses to give is important and demands his presence, but when it is the patient who is scheduled to give information this is a more humble event that requires the attendance of someone on a lower rung of the ladder? Or was there some other reason?

I wanted the consultant to follow my story, listen to my decision and discuss it with me. Although I had so far spent less than an hour in his presence, every minute had been a crucial one because it was contributing to what Brody, in *Stories of Sickness*, calls 'the joint construction of narrative' – the process whereby patients come to physicians with broken stories as much as with broken bodies, and together they construct a narrative that is important precisely because it is a jointly constructed one and the true story of what is happening in the patient's life. Professional and guarded though he was, the consultant had been the co-author of my story up to this point, because the crucial biomedical input was solely his, it was he who had given me life-changing information along my illness route and it was he who had witnessed my responses to it. Through him I felt that the hospital was not just on my side but somehow engaged in my self and my story.

Had he been there for my appointment that afternoon, my consultant would have been able to reflect with me on what had happened during our last meeting, and to respond to the latest development in my story, the moment when I affirmed which of his options I – and therefore he – was going to act upon. Although there had never been any question of him attending my appointment, I felt undermined by his absence, as if I had been presumptuous in expecting a senior figure to take an interest in my junior life and I had a vague sense of not understanding the way things happened in the hospital.

I was beginning to realise something that every patient learns – that arrangements would be made for me, the passive patient, and I would know little about their rationale. Why that particular time? For what particular reason? Why with that particular professional? All kinds of small traditions and shades of power would influence my hospital experience, not just the functional demands of my chosen treatment, and I would have no insight into any of it.

As I sat waiting to see Carys, I felt even more determined to succeed in my mission to be a good patient. I had only fumbled my way through making my decision, but I wouldn't dwell on it. The good patient carries on and is not disheartened. I even began to feel not displeased with my decision and less resentful about being offered a choice, despite the fact that I had been given so little time and information. Now at last I could see the method in this patient choice policy. I had been forced to think through all aspects of the options and to make a decision. As a result, I now had more idea of what my choice of treatment involved, and I had committed myself to it. Sitting in those hospital surroundings, everything seemed simpler than when I was outside the hospital, and all the doubts and worries that had plagued me then now seemed trivial.

My hot hand pressed the steel handle of the door of the breast cancer suite, and I stepped into a room chintzed out with pink and green curtains, pelmet and cushions, all courtesy of the local branch of the Soroptimists, an international service organisation for women in management and the professions. It was like a vibrant stage set that had been transplanted into the stark environment of the NHS hospital. The Soroptimists had sought to make the room less clinical and more domestic, a room where a woman could feel as if she had escaped from the usual spartan hospital surroundings to an environment that recognised her femininity. I felt soothed by the thought that there were other women out there silently offering their support, just as on my previous hospital visit I had been comforted by the poster put up by Bosom Friends.

The room had the same centrepiece as the anteroom where Carys had talked to me immediately after my diagnosis – a teak coffee table with a pink box of paper tissues strategically placed in its centre. Once again I was reminded of the steady procession of women continually going through the same process as me. Tests, diagnosis, prognosis, treatment. Next woman: tests, diagnosis, prognosis, treatment. And, along the way, tears. Carys and I sat facing each other across the coffee table.

'I've decided to have a lumpectomy and radiotherapy', I told her.

'Is that your final decision? On Wednesday you seemed to be going the way of a mastectomy.'

'That was my panic talking. I've thought about it since and read some stuff about it. I've changed my mind about a hundred times, but now I'm definite. Lumpectomy.'

'And you have made your mind up? Is that your final decision?'

Later, when I felt less confident about my decision, I was to think about the way that Carys checked my intentions so thoroughly. I realised that she herself had not expressed any views during the consultation. I never knew her verdict on my choice. I was never clear-sighted enough to ask her, and she never volunteered an opinion.

Now she took a stubby pencil and a sheet of paper and drew a diagram of a breast with its lump and its lymph glands, explaining their significance as she did so. She reminded me that the lump was small. It had breached the wall of the duct where it was growing, so it was an invasive cancer, but it might yet turn out to be grade 1, a mildly aggressive one, and one that had not spread to my lymph nodes, in which case chemotherapy would not be considered appropriate for me.

Chemotherapy. I had been concentrating on the mastectomy versus lumpectomy dilemma and had pushed the possibility of chemotherapy into the dark recesses of my mind. I couldn't remember the consultant even mentioning the word.

Carys continued explaining that all three criteria had to be fulfilled, one or two would not be enough. Small lump, grade 1, and no spread to the lymph nodes. She listed all three alongside the diagram she had drawn of the breast and the lymph glands, and handed me the sheet of paper. I stared at the three phrases and they meant nothing to me. The power of three – all I could think of was the three bears, the three ugly sisters, the three witches in *Macbeth*. All this talk of lymph glands and grades and chemo was alien to me. I wasn't interested. I just wanted it to be over.

Carys looked at me as I sat in the floral cushioned chair. It was a hot, humid day. I was wearing a thin white cotton dress and my dark hair was tied back from my face in an effort to keep cool. Even so, I could feel my cheeks burning and one or two drops of sweat trickling from beneath my armpits. I struggled to take on board the criteria that she had just spelled out. I asked her questions and she went over it all again.

Everything was outside my control. I could do nothing about anything. Was my cancer an aggressive one? I had no idea, but if it did turn out to be aggressive it would alter the whole way in which I thought about myself and my illness, even though my body would feel no different. Had it spread to the lymph nodes in my armpit? I had no idea. Surgeons would scrape out my lymph nodes and send them on to laboratory staff who would look at my cells under a microscope. They would then decide whether the cancer was contained in the breast or had spread to the lymphatic system. So much activity by strangers bent on finding out what was going on underneath my skin.

'I tell you what', said Carys. 'I'll ring the lab and see if they've got the results of your biopsy. I'm allowed to do that – I'm the only nurse with the authority to contact the path lab directly.'

Hardly breathing, I waited while she spoke to a member of staff in the lab. Then she turned to me: 'Good news. It's grade 1 cancer. An excellent result, but we've still got to wait for news about the lymph nodes.'

Having entered the room feeling tense, I now felt nothing but relief and gratitude towards Carys. Her personal authority and charisma allowed her access to information from other departments to which only doctors were privy in the normal way of things. She had managed to get a favourable result for me and it was a lucky sign. Things were not spiralling completely out of control after all.

The medical purpose of my visit had been achieved, and now Carys started to talk about the Welsh village where some of her relatives lived and where my father had been brought up. She moved on to ask me how I was coping with the stress of my diagnosis and what I had told my children. She asked about their reactions. Although I was inside the hospital walls, strands of my outside life and my outside persona were filtering through, and it felt strange. With the exception of my visits to the consultant, I was used to being a one-dimensional patient in the hospital, someone who was looked at only after her hospital notes had been checked over.

Hospital clinics had seemed to me to be places where the patient's individuality and spirituality usually go unrecognised and are suppressed, and where the staff, although they may realise this, are caught up in the daily grind. I could see that Carys was the professional, the nurse specialist, who was going to redress the balance as far as my treatment was concerned. Part of her importance to me was that she didn't have the doctors' kind of expertise. Their expertise was based on having seen many other patients just like me, sorted them and processed them. Carys's expertise was based on looking at my individual case with an open mind and seeking to open out the possibilities of my condition instead of closing them.

What is more, she knew what the doctors really thought. I didn't expect them to be completely open when they were talking to me, the patient, but they would speak their minds to her. Carys would be the link between me and my treatment, my personal narrator, explaining the course of events to me, relating them to my life outside the hospital and, unknowingly, helping me in my quest to maintain my true identity through all the ups and downs of my treatment.

CHAPTER 7

Inpatient

I was a package tourist about to set out on a journey courtesy of the NHS. In exchange for my loss of independence, everything would be arranged for me. The service wouldn't be individually tailored, but it would be economic, convenient and, all being well, trustworthy. However, unlike a holidaymaker, I was only going a few miles down the road, and I was packing my bag in the expectation not of sun and sand but of pain and weakness. I didn't need to pack any daytime clothes, just pyjamas and toiletries, stuff that I associated with early morning and late night, and with the comparatively solitary, dreamy me, not the me of everyday reality.

In that hospital bed I would be a shadow of my everyday self, just a body to be monitored and measured. I would have to fulfil my part of an unspoken contract with the hospital, the part that demands that the good patient be obedient and prepared to give up their independence and control over events. In return I would be given the benefits of modern medicine and technology in order to safeguard my health.

Folding my cotton dressing gown into my small red leather case, I wished that I could keep my right hand from continually feeling for the lump in my breast. I wanted to get my packing over with and forget about this tiny lump and the strange fact that it was now more important than any other part of my body. It overshadowed every single part of my life, and was solely to blame for this dreaded trip to hospital.

Ward 12, my home for the next five days or so, was housed in the same six-storey block as Ward 14, the maternity unit. As I walked from the car park, I could see the window of the room where I had given birth to Ceri 17 years ago. Fourth floor, second window from the left. The labour had proceeded too quickly for a transfer to the delivery room as planned. After the birth was over I was left alone, lying on a high trolley with my tiny baby in a crib next to me. When she cried, instinct took over and I leaned down at a dangerous angle to scoop her up and feed her. Now one of the breasts that had nourished her had turned malignant. Seventeen years ago it had flowed with the vital proteins, minerals and vitamins of breast milk. Now it contained a dry, cancerous lump full of malignant cells. The collision of the two locations, birth ward and breast excision ward, made me feel sentimental and tearful.

Two women in dressing gowns were sitting on a wooden bench just outside the hospital doors, talking loudly, laughing and smoking. The younger one could be no more than thirty, but her face was shadowed and gaunt and her hunched body was barely detectable in its blue quilted wrapping. I had glanced at the reflection of my own face in the mirror before leaving home, seeking signs of illness, but had found none – my eyes were clear, my cheeks pinkish. Unlike the young woman bent over her cigarette, my weight was stable and my body was reasonably full of energy, yet we were both facing grave ill health. 'Patient with serious illness' – she, me and countless others, sharing the same label, although that label had a myriad of different meanings.

Friends and family had focused on me in the past few weeks as someone whose normal life had been suddenly and cruelly interrupted by illness, and there was a part of me that had relished this new role of wounded heroine. As Broyard writes in *Intoxicated by my Illness*, 'Illness is primarily a drama, and it should be possible to enjoy it as well as suffer it.'

Now, here in hospital, illness was humdrum. It had mundane rituals associated with waking, sleeping, eating, ward rounds and medicine rounds. Here I was just another ordinary, everyday patient. Nothing would be expected of me except to exist without causing trouble. After the turmoil of the last few weeks, this passive role had its own appeal. I would be able to relax and leave all of the decisions to the professionals.

Paul strode ahead along the corridor to Ward 12. Used to visiting maternity patients from his practice, he had fallen into his professional doctor role. He greeted a nurse who showed me into my hospital room before disappearing again. After placing my bag on the bed, he started fiddling with a black-and-white television set that balanced on a rickety 1950s-style coffee table. There was a tiny sink on one wall with a mirror above it and a disposal bin next to it. The bed was high and narrow, and when I tested the mattress with my hand I could feel a waterproof layer of thick plastic through the thin undersheet. Another sheet and two thin blankets lay loose on top, not tucked in.

I had once thought that hospital corners – that traditional sheet-tucking method – were a prissy way of making a bed, but now I felt a pang of nostalgia. The staff here didn't care enough for the patients to take the trouble to make their beds comfortable. Then I rallied. This was the NHS in the twenty-first century with its soaring health costs, and I was an able-bodied patient capable of tucking in her own sheets.

Leaning my elbows on the cold brown tiles of the windowsill, I looked at the stick-figures of staff and visitors down below, walking from one building to another. Life was still going on, and I longed to be part of it instead of being trapped in a small high room. I began to resent the pedestrians and their freedom to walk in the open air, to choose their destinations and to take their health for granted, unlike the patients who might be gazing down at them. Then as I stared at them my envy evaporated. Where had it come from? The people I had been glaring at had their own worries and difficulties, and some of them must surely be fellow patients, on their way into or out of the hospital. People just like me.

I opened my case. I had brought three pairs of pyjamas – green and blue stripes, a floral print in shades of purple and green, and a pair printed with pink collie dogs. Bought on a hasty last-minute shopping trip after I'd looked at my usual faded pyjamas with the eyes of a public patient, none of the new ones were to my taste. Now they added to my sense of strangeness as I packed them into the Formica-topped hospital locker. I felt as if I was playing at being a hospital patient. Unlike the previous times I had been admitted to hospital, I was neither feeling ill nor about to give birth.

When I had been admitted to hospital with appendicitis, I was desperate to have the operation as soon as possible so that the inflamed appendix could be sliced out and my pain would disappear. On each of the three occasions when I had gone into hospital to give birth, the pains of labour had ended with the delivery of a new baby.

Now I was having something removed that was not causing any pain. There was going to be no immediate physical gain like the relief of pain or a beautiful new baby. I had to put my faith in doctors and their scientific tests and believe that it was necessary. How I empathised with those women whom I'd read about, who after they find a suspicious lump, put off going to the doctor month after month. They feel healthy and are reluctant to face the possibility of giving up their normal, everyday lives because of one solitary lump and the words of a doctor.

'I'll just put this identification bracelet on you.' A nurse clasped a plastic bracelet with my name inscribed on it around my left wrist, making me feel like a cherished child. The hospital system had decreed that I should wear it, and had created it for me ahead of my arrival. Many members of staff – clerks, nurses and doctors – had exchanged pieces of paper relating to me and my illness, and had worked together behind the scenes to orchestrate my entry into hospital. This narrow plastic band was a sign that I could relax and leave everything to the hospital system.

'Kelly will be coming on duty soon. She's what we call your "named nurse." If you've got any problems, speak to Kelly. She's the one who has overall responsibility for your nursing care and treatment.'

I was relieved. So far a different nurse had entered my room each time. Now I would have someone familiar to watch over me and my treatment and to personally monitor my progress.

When Kelly eventually arrived it was to tell me that she was off duty for the next two days.

'That's a shame. Who will be my named nurse while you're away?'

'No one. I'll catch up with you when I come back. You'll be fine, don't worry.'

I was definitely worried, though, because if the job of named nurse had been deemed necessary, then I wanted one looking after me through the crucial period covering my operation. There didn't seem to be any nurse who assumed managerial responsibility. No senior nurse had appeared or introduced herself to me, and my named nurse had gone. I would be left without a nurse who was taking responsibility for my overall treatment.

Then I remembered that the report sheet was stored at the end of my bed. The nurses were obliged to record all of their measurements and actions on it. It was all down to me now. What a relief. I would be able to monitor things for myself. I would be able to check the items on the report sheet and ensure that everything was going according to plan.

My consultant came into the room to tell me that my operation was scheduled for late the following morning. I stared into his light blue eyes, trying to see through them into his thoughts. This man was making life-and-death decisions on my behalf. Could I be sure he was right? My consultant was the only person taking responsibility for the continuity of my treatment, and I felt new gratitude towards him for that. But would he remove sufficient area around the tumour? Should I be having a mastectomy?

I thought of an anecdote I had once read about Alfred Adler, the psychoanalyst. In 1920, the philosopher Karl Popper had described a case history to him. Adler listened to the account and without any hesitation analysed it in terms of his theory of inferiority feelings. He had never seen the child in question, but he gave a supremely confident judgement. When he had finished, Popper asked him how he could be so sure.

'Because of my thousandfold experience', said Adler.

'And with this new case, I suppose, your experience has become thousand-and-one-fold', said Popper.

Do doctors ever become so complacent that their 'experience' leads them to apply a theory regardless of the nuances of the case before them? Because of his 'experience', my consultant might excise too little flesh, leaving cancer cells behind. He might ignore the signs which indicated that a mastectomy was called for after all.

I thought of the prisoner in Kafka's *The Penal Colony*, who is condemned to be punished by having 'Honour Thy Superiors', the commandment he is deemed to have broken, inscribed ever more deeply into his back. Like him I was powerless. Yet, unlike him, there was no dark threat hanging over me. The superiors who I was now doubting were going to operate to rescue my body, not mutilate it.

Trust. As a good patient I must have complete faith in my doctors and their powers. The doctors owned a wealth of information about my cancer, including observations, measurements and X-rays. My consultant had spent years studying, training and developing expertise. He knew the grade and the cell types of my tumour and other increasingly impenetrable findings. He had investigated hundreds of other breast cancers and could compare and contrast mine in order to be able to fine-tune my treatment. Of course I had faith in him.

Working out how to be a good patient was even more challenging than I had imagined. On the one hand, I did have faith in my consultant, despite my last-minute nerves. On the other hand, how much confidence did I have in the hospital system? I wasn't sure whether I even knew what the system was. I was just a patient, and I had only been in the hospital for a few hours. All I knew was that the system required one person to oversee my medical care, a named nurse, and that I didn't have one – or rather, I did but she had gone. Moreover, Carys, the specialist nurse who I now thought of as my mentor, was on a course and would be unable to visit me during my hospital stay.

What does a good patient do in these circumstances? I would have liked to have left all of the medical monitoring to the professionals. After all, as many experts, including the sociologist Talcott Parsons, have noted, 'a core expectation of being sick is surrendering oneself to the care of a physician.' What is more, the good patient doesn't meddle and isn't so arrogant as to think that she can have a successful input when it comes to her own treatment.

On the other hand, maybe a patient's trust in the hospital system should be an edgy thing – not just a matter of faith, but also based on logic. Since the person responsible for monitoring my treatment had vanished, it would do no harm and might turn out to be useful, might even save me from danger, if after my operation I checked over the report sheets from time to time.

I knew that there was something wrong as soon as I came round in the post-anaesthesia recovery room. My right arm felt as if it had disappeared. I tried to move it, but nothing happened.

A nurse was standing nearby. 'Nurse', I said, 'I can't move my arm.'

She looked over to the other side of the room where the doctor was washing his hands.

'Doctor, she says she can't move her arm.'

He called across 'That's normal. After a breast op there's often some stiffness in the upper arm.'

Stiffness in the arm? My arm was paralysed, not just stiff. I couldn't move it or any of my fingers. They were dead. I felt cold beads of sweat on my forehead. I knew that my arm was paralysed, but I was unqualified to challenge the doctor's claim and his explanation that what I was experiencing was 'normal.' He was the expert, the intellectual link between me and the experiences of countless other patients. He had extensive knowledge. Maybe I was misinterpreting what was happening to me. Maybe the paralysis was similar to paralysis but it was not actual true paralysis, or maybe this kind of paralysis was normal after this particular operation.

I wanted to feel reassured by his words and, sure enough, back in the ward, with the help of a morphine injection, I felt buoyant. My son, Lewis, was the last of the family to visit me. He had jogged the ten miles across the park and streets that lay between his apartment and the hospital. He wore navy tracksuit bottoms and a white singlet on which the words 'Coventry Triathletes' were emblazoned. Hot and larger than life, he flung himself into the black plastic armchair, his sweat glossing the matt black vinyl. His health and energy filled the room so that he seemed to have come from a different planet. Yet as we talked in that strange room, cast in the unfamiliar roles of visitor and bedridden patient, I felt a new kind of communication and intimacy between us that was not merely drug induced.

When I had first entered the hospital I had had a flashback to the time when I had loomed over my passive newborn baby to pick her up. Now my position as a mother was reversed, with my son standing over me, just as Meg and Ceri had done earlier. Now it was I who was lying prone, helpless and dependent, and they who were waiting on me, bringing me essentials that I had forgotten, arranging my pillows and pouring me water.

Illness was giving me the freedom to recognise that I was weak and strong just like them, just like everyone else. I need no longer aspire to be that mythical invincible Welsh mother. But as I lay in my hospital bed recovering from my operation, I had no insight into any shifting dynamics. On the contrary, I felt happy that my relationship with my children was the same as ever. I was the same person, the same mother, and I would persevere in my quest to be a good patient so that things could stay that way.

I didn't mention my paralysed arm to Lewis, Paul or any other members of my family. I didn't even mention it to any of the nurses. It wasn't worth it because it would have recovered by the morning.

CHAPTER 8

Mirrors and masks

As I looked at it, it was no longer my arm, no longer even a part of my body. Instead it had turned into a skin-covered, ashy-pink cylinder that just happened to be lying next to my body. I was desperate to make contact with it. I gathered a handful of the white cotton sheet in my left hand and, eyes shut, passed it across the fingers of my right hand. Was there any sensation? No, I could feel nothing. The cotton sheet was brushing my fingers but my fingers were blind to the cool, coarse texture.

Then once again my brain tried to engage my arm in my intense desire to move it up off the bed. 'Move yourself, arm. Lift yourself up, pl–ea–se.' Nothing happened, no movement.

I felt for the site of the operation on my right breast with my left hand, and was relieved to feel thick cotton wadding covering it. I could forget about that problem for the moment. I remembered a friend telling me about his skiing holiday just before I entered hospital. He said that after he had handed in his skis at the end of the holiday, he did a quick mental audit of his body to check that everything was still working. Now, the morning after my operation, I thought about my changed body and its audit results – a missing chunk of flesh, some missing lymph nodes and a completely lifeless arm.

A nurse came in. 'Morning. Time to get up and wash yourself. I'll put your towel and soap on the locker.' She placed a thin white hospital towel on top of the teak locker next to my bed, and rummaged around inside the locker until she found the pink bar of soap that I had brought in with me. She smacked it down on top of the towel and wheeled around towards the door.

I said quickly 'My arm. I can't move it. I don't think I'll be able to wash myself.'

'You'll be all right once you're up and about', she called.

She was off, having achieved the purpose for which she had entered my room.

What would happen to my dead arm once I was up and about? I would have no sense of where it was or what it was doing – it might swing at an odd angle and it might even break. How would I wash myself or clean my teeth? I started to move myself across to the edge of the bed, only to feel a sudden sharp tug over my right ribs. I opened my pyjama jacket and looked down at my body. There was a tube running from my ribs down the side of the bed to a bottle that stood on the floor, half full of blood. I realised that this was a drain and I would need to carry it with me wherever I went.

The drain was the third constituent of my triple whammy.

First whammy – I had become a patient in a hospital, dependent on the knowledge and technology of the medical staff. I knew nothing about the rationale for anything, what would happen to me next, or who would enter the room next or why.

Second whammy – my paralysed arm was like a dead rabbit hanging at my side. I had to think through every action in advance in order to function with only one hand.

And now third whammy – I would have to carry a drain in my left hand every time I moved, leaving me with no useful hand.

What would a good patient do in these circumstances? My motivation was as strong as ever – if I accomplished my mission to be a good patient, fate would return to me my old life and my old self. But I was becoming agitated. Here in this hospital my skills and knowledge were irrelevant or powerless, so that I couldn't even communicate with the staff. I was faceless, and as for my body, it was fundamentally changed and damaged. Perhaps I should put my quest to one side for the moment and just concentrate on getting through this chaos.

Yes, for now just 'getting through' would be my aim, and in a few days, when I had got a better grip on the situation, I would resume my quest to be a good patient.

I edged myself off the bed to sit on the grey plastic chair next to it, the bottle on the floor beside me and my right arm lying in my lap.

Another nurse entered the room, wheeling a trolley with a machine lying on it. I wondered what it was for and how it was going to help me.

'I just want to measure your blood pressure, dear.'

As she wrapped the cuff around my left arm, I said 'My right arm is paralysed. I can't move it. I can't do anything with it.'

'Hold this arm out, love.' She pointed to the left one.

The machine automatically inflated and deflated the cuff.

The nurse's eyes were fixed on the machine and its reading. I missed the intimacy of the nurse sitting by my side for a few minutes to take my pulse, a nostalgic image remembered from my childhood appendectomy. Electronics had made it redundant.

She said, 'Don't worry, it will be all right. Lots of women have that problem after a breast op. It's because they took some of your lymph nodes.'

She unhooked the machine and left.

The next person to enter the room was in her early twenties and wearing a white tunic and white trousers. She put her clipboard down on the locker.

'Hello, I'm Mandy. I'm a physiotherapist.'

Athletic build, bouncy walk – I should have guessed.

'I've come to give you some exercises for your arm. The arm can be stiff after breast surgery, so you need to work on it with some exercises.'

She asked me to stand next to the wall and then lift my arm up and walk my fingers as far as I could up the wall. She demonstrated with her own young healthy arm. 'Now you do it', she said.

'I can't. Something has happened to my arm. I can't move it or my fingers.'

'That's what these exercises are for', Mandy said, intent on working her way through her standard protocol. 'Lift your arm up and walk your fingers like this.'

I used my left hand to grasp my right forearm and pull it up next to the wall and then to push it up further, so that my dead fingers coasted upwards along the pale green paint.

'Hm', Mandy said, frowning. She paused for a few moments, then briefly wrote on her clipboard and handed me a leaflet that illustrated three impossible arm exercises. Then she left to go through the same procedure with her next patient.

New to her job, she was uncomfortably aware that she had not yet reached the stage of accommodating patients who didn't fit into her protocol. I knew how she felt because I, too, was dismayed by the way in which my lifeless arm had its own power to interrupt what should have been the normal course of my recovery.

The challenges of being a hospital patient were building up thick and fast. Although I was at first pleased to be in a single room, now I regretted that I wasn't in a ward with other patients from whom I could glean information about the staff and the daily routines. There I wouldn't have to decipher everything for myself and I would have some warning of the approach of all the different professionals. They would walk across the wide room, maybe speak to another patient first, and I would be able to watch and learn and speculate about the purpose of their visits. I would also have a few minutes to prepare myself in order to explain to them about my arm so that they would listen to me.

As it was, the staff visits to my small room were sudden, unannounced and brief, and I felt as if I was telling them about my arm with a ghost voice that I could hear but they could not. Perhaps it was because my personal knowledge about my paralysed arm hadn't been validated by any technology or any medical opinion. It was a kind of 'subjugated knowledge', 'naive' and 'located low down on the hierarchy, beneath the required level of cognition or scientificity', as described by Foucault in *Health and Medicine*.

My interactions with the staff left me in no doubt about their concept of a 'good' patient, and it fitted in with my decision to 'just get through' my treatment. Most of the time I found myself behaving in a process that Anselm Strauss has described in *Mirrors and Masks*:

> Everyone presents himself to others and to himself, and sees himself in the mirrors of their judgements. The masks he then

and thereafter presents to the world and its citizens are fash-
ioned upon his anticipations of their judgements.

It was best to mirror the staff's expectations, and to be polite, trusting and
obedient. It was best to wear a mask – to reveal no opinions and show no
emotion. And it was best not to ask too many questions. Questions would
slow staff members down and leave less time for other patients.

Mid-morning, my consultant arrived. Yet again I tried to tell a health
professional that my arm and hand no longer worked. This time my
words fell upon fertile ground, partly because the consultant was well
enough acquainted with me to recognise the panic in my voice, and
partly because his scientific antennae were alert to symptoms of all kinds
and to their meaning over the passage of time.

I said 'My arm just swings from my shoulder. I've got no control over it.'

He nodded. 'Yes, I've noticed that.'

I felt as if someone had reactivated the talk button on my voice volume
control.

'And my hand is paralysed.'

'Can you move your fingers?'

He demonstrated how he would like me to bend and stretch the fingers
on my right hand. Then we both stared at my impotent fingers. They
wouldn't move, not even for a doctor.

The consultant looked at me and was silent. It felt like the moment after
my diagnosis when he had done nothing and said nothing, but just shared
the moment with me, just respected and recognised my distress.

Eventually he said 'This is baffling. But don't worry, I'll get back to you
on this.'

Paul was the last visitor of the morning, and had come straight from his
surgery. He frowned when he saw that I was still not using my arm. He
asked me to try to move my fingers.

'Move your fingers, idiot' I urged myself, but my fingers just lay there,
deaf and lifeless.

'Don't worry', Paul said. 'It's a neurological thing. Nerve damage of
some sort. But don't worry – nerves can regenerate and grow. You'll get
the control back.'

Yes, I would. I was determined about that.

Paul topped up the water in my vases and gave me my pills to swal-
low. With only one working hand, I had been unable to pop them out
of their foil containers.

'I can't seem to get through to the nurses the fact that my arm is paralysed.'

'That's because they know that breast cancer patients normally have
some stiffness of the upper arm after the operation, because the lymph
nodes have been cut out. They just don't realise that that isn't what you're
talking about.'

His eyes fell on the yogurt pot that contained part of my lunch. He removed the foil lid so that I could at last get at its contents. Then his gaze wandered round the room looking for any other sign of unfulfilled need.

'I'll be back later on after evening surgery. Don't worry, it will be all right.'

He patted my shoulder, just as my doctor had done earlier. At the door he turned, came back and leant over to kiss me.

In the early evening he returned carrying a blue plastic box. During his earlier visit my face had started twitching – a temporary side-effect, he had reassured me, of the operation. Now he opened the box to reveal some cheese straws that he had cooked that afternoon. He'd added extra salt to the cheese straws and spread them with a highly salted meat extract spread, a favourite food of mine despite its dubious origins.

'I think the problems with your face might be due to lack of salt or magnesium' he said.

'If you eat some of these it will top your level up again.'

I bit into a cheese straw and flaky crumbs cascaded over the floor. About 30 minutes later my face began to grow still and the muscles relaxed.

Who would have thought that cheese straws could make a romantic offering? The mix of the medical and domestic, the right minerals housed in comfort food, was a beguiling remedy. I was conscious that an element of the patient–doctor duality was creeping into our relationship, but it was all right because it was a mild and tender version of it.

Things were looking up. Paul had given me hope that my arm and hand would eventually recover, and at last a member of the hospital staff, my consultant, had recognised the fact that my arm and hand were indeed paralysed.

Ever since the operation, my breast under its thick cotton dressing had no longer been at the top of my list of worries. Presumably the lump and its environs had been removed, along with an unspecified number of lymph nodes from under my arm, and I would have to wait to hear whether or not the cancer had spread to my lymph nodes. This worry was a dull, thudding ache, but for the moment it was pushed into second place by my catastrophic hand.

I had lost my second most vital tool, my right hand. It would have been my first but, luckily, I was left-handed. On the other hand, playing the piano, writing, cooking, driving and so on all required my active right hand. Without it I would be a different person, unable to do the activities that defined me, although for now I was in limbo, protected from the full reality of my loss by my role as a passive patient.

I had come into hospital to be operated on for breast cancer, a story that everyone – medical professionals, friends and relatives – could understand. Now there was a subplot to the story, a paralysed arm that was not in the original script. It was not my fault, but even so there was something wayward about entering hospital for treatment for a life-threatening disease and then adding another unrelated problem en route. Had this happened to any other patients? How had it happened?

I found myself missing Gaia, my Internet muse, the magical being who would normally answer my questions. She could be trusted to unearth the facts as well as their colourful contingencies, including the dubious and the discredited. I wanted to find out information for myself when I most needed it, as well as to be told the pure facts as selected by the experts in their own time.

CHAPTER 9

Aftercare

It was Saturday, so he was dressed casually – pale blue denim shirt and cream-coloured slacks – but he still looked like a harassed consultant. I was sitting up in bed staring at the limp arm lined up next to me. Without the paralysis I would have been up and about and almost back to normal. The consultant, too, stared at my arm.

'I spent last night looking up my medical textbooks. It seems that the problem is that the radial nerve has been crushed and that's the cause of the lack of movement of the arm and hand.'

'Oh, right ... thanks for finding that out.'

'One of the usual causes is prolonged pressure on the nerve from the position of the arm during sleep or coma.'

'Is it something that happens often?'

'It's extremely unusual. The classic example is of a drunk who develops it after going to sleep with his arm draped tightly over a chair. It becomes more and more crushed by the chair, and the radial nerve is compressed.'

'So how did my injury happen?'

He tugged at a handful of his brown curls.

'Your injury must have occurred during surgery, I'm afraid. I'm very sorry about that.'

'I'm in good company then. Me and a comatose drunk.'

Although he tried to smile at my attempt at humour, his lips barely moved.

'I would expect you to regain the complete use of your arm and hand within the next three months.'

He sighed. It was probably not him but a nurse or anaesthetist who had pinned back my arm in readiness for the operation. My injury was of the accidental kind, and anyway, as a consultant, in this kind of situation he was probably accountable to no one but himself. Yet he was holding himself professionally responsible for the accident, and had spent his spare time researching the problem of my arm.

He was a man of few words, with a reputation for being distant, but to me he was a recognisable type of doctor – the kind that you can understand more if you are open to what they do rather than to what they say.

We stared at each other and it seemed to me that there was a kind of connection between us, as if we recognised each other's unspoken worries.

Then he said 'Is there anything else you want to know? Anything about your operation?'

Immediately I thought of my lymph nodes. Were they cancerous or not? I was desperate to know, but I instantly ruled out mentioning them because it was too early. I had been told that I would be given the results of the operation three weeks after surgery. It was no good asking the consultant. He was part of the system and was only allowed to divulge information at the appointed time. So I didn't ask him.

He picked up the drain bottle and looked at its bloody contents.

'They haven't marked the level', he said. 'Bad.'

A nurse had forgotten to record the blood level not only on that day but also the previous day. The consultant had no idea of the rate at which blood was draining out of my wound. My drain would have to remain in longer than he had estimated, he told me with a resigned shake of the head, and I wouldn't be able to be discharged until the following day.

'Very bad', I said.

Three days ago I had been relieved to see that my report sheet was stored at the end of my bed. In the absence of my named nurse who would have overseen the records, I myself would be able to check and ensure that everything was going according to plan. Now it was obvious that my strategy had failed due to my lack of medical knowledge. It had never occurred to me that it was necessary to measure the volume of blood seeping out of the drain. My one small attempt at mustering some control of my treatment had failed.

I thought of an article I had once read that had been an influence on my original decision to check on my notes. It had been written by a journalist who had recently been discharged from hospital after extended treatment for a serious illness. The article described how at one stage she had been unable to discourage a nurse who insisted on hooking up another bottle of her infusion at a speed that might have burst her veins. After the nurse had left, the writer changed the volumetric pump to a slower drip.

'I learned that the safest thing in hospital is to learn how to do things yourself', she wrote.

She had acted as a maverick expert patient. There are some official expert patients around – patients who have been trained to be key decision makers in their own treatment. The notion of the expert patient is based on the theory that in the case of chronic illness, patients and professionals each have their own area of knowledge and expertise and need to work together.

The journalist and I were the underground, untrained versions of the expert patient, improvising covertly in areas not envisaged by the professionals. The journalist had become well versed over time in the routines of transfusions, and her venture was successful. I was a novice, experiencing everything for the first time and, despite the modest monitoring task I had set myself, I had failed. What would the good patient have done? Would she have left well alone? After all, institutions must have rules or anarchy would reign. Alternatively, would the good patient have mugged up on all the daily minor medical procedures before she went into hospital so that she had the necessary knowledge to safeguard her own treatment?

Now I was upset and confused, and unsure what to do next. I was ready to resume my mission to be a good patient, but it was not turning out to be easy. Yes, I wanted to be a good patient, but in whose eyes?

'I know someone who had a paralysed hand and arm just like yours after surgery.'

My cousin, Nia, drew up a chair next to me.

'She was at school with me. I remember she was absolutely terrified that she would never ever be able to use them again.'

'What happened? Was she all right?'

'It took some time, but eventually she got the use of them back. She went completely back to normal and started playing tennis again. She could use her arm and her hand just as well as before.'

I saw myself through Nia's eyes as someone who was only temporarily disabled, only temporarily a patient, and this gave me new hope. I realised that I had started to feel as if I would be stuck in this patient role for ever. Instead I would be like Nia's friend and return to my old life.

There is nothing so encouraging as anecdotal evidence from friends. All the reassurances of Paul and the doctor, based on real medical evidence, were nothing compared with this real-life example, albeit a second-hand one. Someone I knew had witnessed someone they knew recover from the very same paralysis that I had. Nia had witnessed someone who had suffered the same fears as me, and she had witnessed her complete recovery and return to normal life. I could soon be like her friend, arm recovered and treatment over.

After Nia had left, the converse images of her friend with a limp arm and then, months later, using it to wave a tennis racket around lingered in my mind and often resurfaced to reassure me in the coming weeks.

Soon afterwards, Emily, the nurse, came in carrying a two-handled cotton bag printed with vivid red roses and emerald green leaves.

'This is to put your drain in', she said. 'Makes it easier to carry it around. Bosom Friends make them.'

'Is that the Bosom Friends from around here?'

She hovered by the door on her way out.

'Bosom Friends? Yes, they're a local support group. They've all had what you've got and they do things like this. Help women with breast cancer.'

I stared at the bag. Its scarlet and emerald colours glowed against the pastel-painted walls of my cell. Running my left hand along the coarse cotton material, I felt small neat stitches bump beneath my fingers. They were the work of women who had been operated on for breast cancer, and they were signalling the women's support in the same way as their poster in the hospital corridor when I was waiting for my diagnosis.

I flopped down on the bed. Out of bed I was continually aware of the limp weight of my arm.

'There's a Bosom Friend outside to see you. Do you want her to come in?'

Emily was balanced on one foot with her upper body draped round the door, her blonde head leaning into the room.

'Yes', I said, although I wasn't sure I was up to meeting a stranger.

A woman who had neat brown hair and was wearing a navy blazer and cream skirt came and sat on the chair next to my bed, avoiding eye contact. 'I'm Ruth from Bosom Friends. How are you?'

I didn't want to confuse the issue by talking about my disabled hand and arm when her speciality was breast cancer.

'I'm getting on quite well. I can't believe how quickly everything has happened.'

'When were you diagnosed?'

'Just three weeks ago.'

'My husband has prostate cancer. He was diagnosed six months ago and he's still waiting for the date for his surgery.'

I felt as if I had been tactless, and we sat in silence for a while. Things were not going well. Why should they? Bosom Friends was an amateur organisation, a team of women with breast cancer doing their best for other women with breast cancer.

'She ran the London Marathon while she was still having her chemo.'

I realised that Ruth had started talking again. 'Sorry, who was that?'

'A friend of mine, Marina. As soon as she came out of hospital after her mastectomy, she started her training.'

'How did she do it?'

'She started by doing just two miles a day, and she gradually built up.'

Suddenly Ruth and I were talking on the same wavelength. We had both had operations for breast cancer and both faced the fact that our bodies were vulnerable. I was inspired by the story of Marina's athletic achievement and by Ruth's own story as well – she herself had qualified as an aerobics instructor a few months after her treatment.

I had lived in that hospital room for three days and not once thought about the power and capacity of my body. I realised that I had caved in and thought of it as an invalid body, in every respect. I had accepted my infirmity too easily, and it was time to resume my active quest to be a good patient. What was a damaged breast, a limp arm in the vast human catalogue of injuries? I had let them take over my view of myself too easily.

After Ruth had left, I positioned myself next to the bed. I held the bag with the drain in it in my left hand and started jogging. After a while I turned round and saw myself in the large mirror on the wall above the washbasin. A dark-eyed woman with pale skin and black, shoulder-length hair looked back at me. Her right arm dangled by her side. She was wearing a pink dressing gown and held a shopping bag that was covered with deep red roses. A plastic tube was just visible as it emerged from under her pyjama top and disappeared into the bag. A strange sight, but Ruth's visit had reminded me that I was normal. There were tribes of women in my situation, achieving all kinds of things and not taking themselves or their illnesses too seriously.

The next day, just before I was discharged from hospital, Kelly, my named nurse, returned.

'How are you? Did everything go well for you?'

My paralysed arm was a surprise to her because it was not written up in my notes.

'That's awful – tell me all about it', she said.

'Tell me all about it.' No medical professional had said those gratifying words to me since I visited the consultant for the first time in Rushwood Hospital.

It became obvious that the withdrawn Kelly whom I had first met, who had told me that she, my named nurse, would be deserting me, had been feeling some guilt about this even though it was the system's fault, and not hers, that I had been left without a named nurse. She massaged my inert hand while I talked, she listened carefully and she even asked questions to encourage me to expand my story further. I saw myself through her eyes as a person with feelings instead of just a body with a disease to be medically treated.

It was a bittersweet experience because now I knew exactly what I had missed by not having a named nurse. I could have had 'my' nurse in the same way as I had 'my' consultant. Someone who might have listened long enough to realise that my arm was paralysed, and who would have checked that all measurements were being recorded. Someone who might have taken a day-to-day interest in my ups and downs and known the real story of my hospital stay – its events, the main characters and how I felt about it all.

I was one of the many inpatients who are in hospital for only a few days, with little time to build up relationships with the busy staff. The named nurse system was designed to overcome this problem. The theory was right although the practice had failed in my case. Well, the good patient accepts inevitable imperfections in the hospital system and does not dwell on the past. No named nurse, but I had received post-operative care of diverse kinds and in varying degrees from many other sources – medical and lay, official and unofficial.

My overworked left hand jammed my clothes and toiletries into my red leather case as I got ready to take my leave. Four days previously I had been admitted to hospital to have an operation to remove my tumour, its environs, and the lymph nodes from under my right arm, and this had all been successfully achieved. Now it was time to regain control of my life.

CHAPTER 10

Disconnected

Meg lifted my right hand on to the piano keyboard and slid the battered pages of the piano solo version of 'Rhapsody in Blue' on to the music shelf.

'Try it', she said.

Then I knew that she shared my thoughts. I had arrived home from hospital that afternoon and the time was ripe to jump-start my hand. The touch of my fingers on the cold, smooth keys would revitalise the connection with my brain. The memory of all those years of practise, of scales and arpeggios and sonatas, would jolt my fingers into action. The connection with my brain was still there – it just needed a musical stimulus to reset itself.

Nothing happened. My fingers lay like small blocks of lead on the keys.

I turned to Meg. 'The radial nerve in my arm is still out for the count.'

'Have another go, Mum.'

Concentrated silence.

Eventually I gave up and played the melody line of the opening four bars with my left hand, hearing not the thin sounds of the piano notes but the raw power of the wailing clarinet of the original version.

'Well', I said, 'I suppose it's no use crying over a hopeless hand.'

'Your nerve will wake up eventually and reconnect your hand with your brain. That's what Dad said anyway.'

'Yes, and then I'll be back to normal. Just a matter of time.'

'Definitely', Meg said. 'Let's go in the kitchen and I'll make you a cup of tea.'

Leaning against the cool tiles of the kitchen counter, I stared out into the street. A group of young schoolchildren were on the pavement outside our house. One was swinging on a low branch of the tall oak tree, and the others were swiping at its branches with their rucksacks as they made their way home from their last day of school. On the other side of the road Angie was hurrying her eight-year-old son into her car to take him to his karate class.

The kitchen window was like a thick, impenetrable glass screen, allowing me to view normal life even though I was stuck in another country – illness country. Mammograms, scans, drips and scars – these were the stuff of illness country. The people outside my window went about their everyday lives mostly unmindful of the vulnerability of their bodies unless they had an illness. I had become a patient, used to fear, relief, fear – the cycle of emotions that related to the hidden messages of my body.

Unlike those normal people in the outside world, I was totally immersed in my body and its current state. I kept thinking about the pink scar pointing from under my armpit across my chest and wondering about what was happening underneath it. Were cancer cells milling around, eager to spread themselves? I was stuck, a patient who still felt allied with the hospital staff, and whose future was dependent on the test results they would give me in two weeks' time.

At some stage in the past few weeks I had passed into illness territory. I sat and looked around my kitchen. It was still the same – the same cooker, the same oak table, there was even a dull green pepper inside the fridge that had been shrivelling there ever since I went into hospital – but now it all seemed like a stage set. It was my kitchen, but I felt like a ghost in it.

Although I was home from hospital, I was still in that other country that Susan Sontag calls 'the kingdom of the sick.' I had felt in limbo in hospital and had looked forward to returning home, like an emigrant pining to return to the old country. But now it seemed that illness wasn't just a matter of geography, and the journey home from hospital had not restored me to normality.

My identification bracelet was still on my left wrist. Unable to chop it off with my useless right hand, I had still not got round to asking anyone else to do it. I sat at the table and kept scraping the bracelet's plastic edge across my numb right hand, obsessively trying to provoke a response.

I gave up, and picked up a magazine that Meg had been reading earlier. Flicking with one hand through its fashion pages, I noticed that my body with its scar and paralysed arm had crept far outside the beauty world's norms. The message was that women should have control over their bodies come what may, and there were advertisements and features selling beauty products, plastic surgery or dieting aids. Each, of these, or any combination of them, could be relied upon to get one's own faulty body back on the right track so that it fitted into the kind of glamorous world that the magazine portrayed. Once I had found this carrot-and-stick approach to bodily control and self-improvement darkly entertaining, but now it seemed more dark than entertaining.

The magazine's cold and impersonal consumerist eye was giving me the same helpless feeling that I had experienced when I first met my consultant in Rushwood Hospital for my initial tests. Here was the same objective gaze that could judge the unknown me and fail me. Many weeks ago, I had wanted my consultant to look at me as an individual, not as a one-dimensional patient. I had wanted him to see me as someone whose history was rooted within the friendly contexts of family and community. Now I was experiencing the same feeling of being one-dimensional that I had felt then. Morris identifies the cause of this kind of unease as follows: 'In a culture dominated by the vision of utopian bodies, illnesses that twist and distort the human figure will register as vaguely disreputable signs of personal defeat.'

Fresh from hospital, I was confronted with the realisation that in the outside world, a body could be considered defective and in need of correction even though it was perfectly healthy. I was back home, but everything seemed changed and nothing seemed normal.

'Phone for you, mum.' Meg brought the phone and put it in my left hand.

It was Emma. 'It's bad news', she said. 'Carys, the Breast Care nurse, is leaving. She's got a job in a London teaching hospital. Everybody's upset about it.'

Carys was a vital person in my treatment – the link between home and hospital. I knew that I could ring her at any time. I had never done so, but just knowing that I could was like a golden thread between me and the hospital. Carys couldn't just go and desert me at this crucial time.

'She leaves at the end of next week', Emma said, 'and there's a party at the hospital tomorrow. It's in the Staff Social Club. You know it – that battered old Nissan Hut at the far side of the hospital. I'll pick you up at noon.'

It was my first time out since my hospital discharge, but the prospect was less daunting than it would normally have been, because I would be meeting fellow patients.

In a dingily lit bar that had a slight odour of disinfectant, we sat at long wooden tables on which there were jugs of orange juice and platters of assorted sandwiches and cakes. There were over a hundred of us – women of all ages from young mothers with toddlers to a group of smartly dressed women in their eighties – and almost all of us had been operated on for breast cancer at some stage in our lives.

The women sitting around me sounded pleased that Carys's talents had been recognised in the shape of a higher-level job and a hefty rise in salary. Even so, many of them murmured agreement when a woman with sharp cheekbones and shadowed eyes sitting nearby said 'I thought of Carys as a friend. I'd forgotten that she's a professional woman with a career.'

She sounded slightly resentful and I knew why. Like me, she'd come to depend upon Carys as the constant throughout her treatment, always available to explain and give advice as needed.

Carys's role in the hospital had been unique in a way that few other nurses could aspire to, and that the doctors never could because they were too distanced by their primary involvement in the biological science of our disease. Carys's personal charisma and wide knowledge of the effects of cancer and cancer treatment had earned her unique authority and trust among her patients, especially since we knew that she had nursed both her mother and her sister through terminal cancer.

Jo, the single mother of a four-year-old boy, told us that she had been diagnosed a few days after Christmas the previous year. When she had had a panic attack during the night of New Year's Eve, she had phoned Carys.

'I was terrified I wouldn't live to see my little boy grow up. We're so close, and he'd be completely lost without me. I was scared out of my wits. But Carys was wonderful to me.'

Besides making herself accessible to her patients out of hours, Carys had set up Bosom Friends, the support group which included in its ranks Emma, Samira Khan (whom I'd met at Rushwood Hospital) and Ruth (my bedside visitor). In a brief speech, Carys reassured us that she wouldn't lose touch but would make frequent return visits to the hospital and to Bosom Friends.

We drank a toast to her, and as I raised my glass with my left hand the sleeve of my navy jacket fell back. The eyes of the woman sitting opposite rested on my identification bracelet.

'Oh look. You've still got your identity band on. Has anyone got any scissors?'

The word went round, but mercifully no one had a pair of scissors and I kept my left arm down so that the band was hidden once more.

Then Carys came over, her dark eyes glancing over the women sitting around the trestle table.

'Who wants a pair of scissors?'

'She does.' The woman opposite pointed at me. 'They forgot to take her identity band off.'

Carys looked at my pink face.

'Shall I cut if off?'

'Might as well.'

Her scissors snipped and she put the plastic relic into my outstretched left hand.

'I'm glad I was here to see you out of hospital', she said. 'Good luck with the rest of your treatment.'

With Carys's departure went the personal link with the hospital that had meant so much to me. Now I felt even more dependent on my family and friends. When visitors arrived, my post-operative lethargy disappeared and I needed little encouragement to tell them all that had happened to me. They were witnesses to my disordered state but they were also my interpreters, and I saw my illness partly through their eyes.

My account of my illness improved as I retold it, becoming more polished and narrative. Parts of the story that were unclear or meandering, I reflexively sharpened up depending on the personality of the visitor and how well I knew her. After the shock and silence of the past weeks I was trying out new voices, new ways of being myself, but through them all ran a strand of desperation because I was also trying to rehabilitate myself in my friends' eyes. I was trying to present myself as a cool-headed patient, efficient and in control of events – a 'good' patient.

To a friend who was stolid and practical, I emphasised my competence as my illness unfurled, and gave her a straightforward, unemotional account of what had happened, including how I had looked everything up on the Internet and therefore knew what to expect from the medics.

A droll neighbour was given a humorous account of the difficulties that my dangling hand and arm had got me into in the hospital.

Those who spoke in hushed voices as if I was doomed were treated to an over-emphatic explanation relating to my cancerous lump and its small dimensions.

'The cancer was in the very early stages,' I told them. 'It was caught in time.'

These were two sentences that I had heard others use successfully to put an end to speculation, and they emerged automatically from my lips like mantras.

I told this ever changing story to a series of listeners, and after a time I could hear my voice sounding inauthentic even as I spoke. Inauthenticity is a way of living that lacks self-awareness, according to the philosopher, Heidegger, and it is rooted in our absorption in the ways of living that others exemplify. The individual's view of herself and her life arises from what 'they' think is good and what 'they' think is normal. Of course, most of us are happy to follow the routines and fashions of those around us for much of the time, because it would be unfeasible to constantly reinvent ways of living, but now I was taking this everyday sociability to an extreme.

Newly out of hospital and struggling to return to my 'normal' identity, I had been relating my story to my visitors while all the time bearing in mind 'they' values and 'they' ways of behaving and speaking. I had had one eye on my story and one eye on what others expected of me. Others, it seemed to me, saw me as a patient and a victim who had lost control, so I must struggle against this stereotype. Therefore I tailored my story to each visitor so as to present myself as someone who was in supreme control of her life.

It was a simple question that visitors never failed to ask that saved me from my headlong trip into phoniness. I became increasingly beguiled by the polite enquiry 'How *are* you?', delivered in that particular tone which some patients find irritating – the gently sympathetic tone with the emphasis on '*are*' that people reserve for those with serious illness. Completely unlike the routine enquiry of everyday bonhomie, it recognised me as vulnerable.

Critical illness, wrote Anatole Broyard in *Intoxicated by my Illness*, is 'like a great permission ... all your life you think you have to hold back your craziness, but when you're sick you can let it out in all its garish colours.' Where once I had been afraid of revealing myself, now I had an obvious weakness that was impossible to hide. I had received the right to be vulnerable – and in public, too. Moreover, friends indicated that they felt closer to me because they knew that I had faced my own death. I felt myself relaxing into the idea that the depths and dissonances of my life could be revealed to others. I would retain my dignity and they wouldn't reject me.

The 'great permission' that illness offered me also suffused my relationships with my children. The nature of my connection with them had been changing ever since they visited me as I lay helpless in my hospital bed. I had come out of hospital, arm dangling and literally 'disarmed', and whenever the children were around they waited on me with cups of coffee and cooked meals, and chauffeured me to various destinations. My illness had been a turning point. Turning points, as defined by Bruner, 'represent a way in which people free themselves in their self-consciousness from their history.'

He points out that it is unsurprising that turning points occur at moments when the culture gives more freedom. Forced by illness into dependency, I had been freed from my own rigid conception of motherhood, as well as what I believed to be others' expectations of me as a mother. Implicit in my changing relationship with the children had grown the acknowledgement that I, too, was vulnerable just like them, just like everyone else. My role of patient had given me the opportunity to abandon my old conception of motherhood, to set myself free from my 'strong mother' role and to recognise the nuances of a new kind of communication and a new kind of identity. It hadn't happened all at once or even completely, for my original construct of being a 'good' mother would always be part of me.

I had loved being a 'Welsh mother.' It had been my ambition since I was a little girl, even before that visit when I had confided in the school inspector, and there was a delight and exhilaration in the role and its raw femininity and power. But now illness had zoomed in on its weaknesses, and my identity as a mother was shifting and dissolving into a more profound and egalitarian concept.

Yet even as my role was changing during those first weeks out of hospital when everything seemed so unreal, I was in denial. The changes in my relationships with the children were just the temporary ones of illness. My illness was just an interruption before I returned to my old life and my old familiar role of mother. All the changes that I was facing, including Carys's imminent departure, made it even more essential that I had a vision of future peace and normality to support me.

It was a huge temple filled with plants and flowers as well as greetings cards, ornaments, clothes, sweets and biscuits. Just a week after my return from hospital and, as a distraction from my avid desire to learn my pathology results, a close friend had invited me to accompany her on an expedition to our local garden centre. On the way there I had told Rachel how worried I was about my results and given her a detailed run-down of my tumour, its characteristics and the further findings that the results might uncover.

Once we were at the garden centre, none of the extensive ranges of merchandise distracted me from my fixation. When we took a break in the café area for a coffee and a cheese salad, I kept talking about my lymph nodes and what Carys had told me relating to them. Around us other women were sitting relaxed, exchanging snatches of conversation. I was leaning hyperactively across the table towards Rachel, giving her no chance to change the subject. I felt like a puppet and my fears about my illness were pulling the strings. I muttered on and on in a trajectory of isolated despair, and Rachel, being a good friend, listened.

Our shopping completed, we were about to leave when a friend of Rachel's appeared. I gestured that I would wait by the exit while they talked.

I stepped outside and stared at the vast grey sky, feeling physically drawn into its infinite depths. Slowly I began to feel its power and benevolence. I became aware of the millions of people who had already lived on this earth who seemed to be at one with the sky above. I could feel and almost see their presence in its grey depths. The sky seemed deep with sadness and joy and the presence of past and present souls, and it was in unity with them. All of us inside and outside that garden centre, whoever we were, were part of the great eternal cosmos. We were nothing and everything. We belonged to the past, the present and the future.

Afterwards, I stood holding my potted plant feeling completely disorientated. I felt as if I had undergone a spiritual experience. But in a garden centre? Around me were people pushing trolleys loaded up with plants and oddments. Not the sort of venue conducive to mystic occurrences. What was happening to me?

The vision mirrored the one that I had experienced just after the consultant had given me my diagnosis. Then the recognition of the infinite depths and heights and the full spectrum of humanity inherent in the blue sky outside the tiny consulting room had calmed me. I had later learned from Gaia that this kind of experience is referred to as a 'vision', and that many people have mystical visions like this. They confirm our essential humanness and are especially likely to be experienced during illness, with its attendant stress and emotion.

When I think back to my visions, I feel again the joy, the sadness, the resignation, the hope and, above all, the peace of life and death, and I feel again the awesome sense of communion with others. It was as if my visions were binding me to being human and being part of an infinite whole in the face of disconnection and bodily disruption. At the time, an ordinary commercial English garden centre had seemed an almost comic venue for experiencing such a vision. Only later did it strike me that its very commonplace nature made it an apt location, not a comic one at all.

On the way home, I turned towards Rachel, noticing her strong classical features and her golden hair twined into a loose knot for what felt like the first time that day. She had lost her husband, Jeff, to cancer just a year previously, but even so she had paid attention to my obsessive talk about cancer throughout the afternoon. She stared at the road ahead, as if we were still on the timeless journey of my vision.

'Thanks, Rachel.'

'For what?'

'For not telling me to shut up when I was going on about my lymph nodes.'

She laughed. 'Don't worry. Just say what's on your mind. You'll be all the better for it.'

CHAPTER 11

Predictions

Sometimes I still thought of the future with my old supposition that I would live to my eighties. Other times I saw life only a few months ahead and a gauze curtain hanging down, blurring the rest of it. Was I going to live a normal life? Was I going to die within the next few years? My agonising was compulsive but at the same time deeply boring. I longed for the day when I would return to Parkside Hospital to meet with my oncologist and hear the results of my tests. Then the misery of waiting would be over and I would know my prognosis. Had the cancer spread? If so, what was in store for me? If it hadn't, how likely was it to spread in the future?

Restless and urgent, I read a poem by the American poet, Jane Kenyon. In 'Prognosis', the walker in the woods expresses her desperate longing to know the future:

Prognosis

I walked alone in the chill of dawn
while my mind leapt, as the teachers

of detachment say, like a drunken
monkey. Then a gray shape, an owl,

passed overhead. An owl is not
like a crow. A crow makes convivial

clucking as it flies,
but the owl flew well beyond me

before I heard it coming, and when it
settled, the bough did not sway.

My mind, too, had been leaping wildly like the 'drunken monkey' of the poem, but now I was enthralled by the image of the silent owl flying in expansive, undefined space beyond the lonely walker. The owl is the embodiment of the future, and Kenyon's walker in the woods is unable to track its passage and is unnerved by that inability. I, too, needed a forecast of the future in order to gain hope and certainty. And as part of my quest to be a good patient, I also needed to avoid introspective anxiety and heed 'the teachers of detachment.' Returning to the poem again and again during this waiting time, I found that it shared and validated my fears and gave me a passing kind of calm.

Seeking clues about my future, I once more became obsessed with Gaia, my Internet muse, just as I had been when I had first discovered my lump. At my meeting with Carys, my nurse specialist, just after I had first been diagnosed, she had told me that the underarm lymph nodes were crucial in a cancer prognosis. I now searched through all the cancer sites in 'My Favourites', seeking further information on this topic. Eventually my worries zoomed in on two questions. Had the cancer already spread to the lymph nodes under my arm? And if it had, how badly did this affect my prognosis?

I was learning about cancer on an unscientific, 'need-to-know' basis rather than in a linear, logical way, but at least I was learning about the crucial issues that the oncologist would cover when he gave me my prognosis. I would have an idea of their relative importance and what questions to ask if necessary.

Internet surfing was making me anxious. It reminded me of what a friend had said about the other kind of surfing: 'Standing up on the surfboard isn't easy – the board's on swirling water and it's a challenge just to keep going.' My quest for knowledge was based on an uncertain foundation – my limited medical knowledge. Yet despite my lurching anxieties, when I was sitting in front of my computer I felt more purposeful and more in control than when I was pursuing any other activity, and Gaia, unlike the hospital staff, would always be there to help me.

A prognosis and the way in which the doctors arrived at it had always seemed to me to be a mystical process, but Gaia – not for the first time – deconstructed a medical ritual for me. A 'prognosis', I learned, is basically the doctors' educated guess at how the patient is expected to do after a disease has been diagnosed, based on factors such as stage of disease, kind of disease, response to treatment, age and general state of health.

Next time Emma visited, I checked this out with her.

'Yes', she said. 'My consultant told me that statistics only tell us what happens to most people. They can't tell us what will happen to the individual. An illness might be 90% fatal, but if you're in the lucky 10% it's not fatal, full stop. The doctor can't be absolutely certain about the outcome for a particular patient.'

'That makes prognosis a dodgy thing for the doctor', I said.

'Yes, he has to be sensitive and if it's bad news, work out how much bad news the individual patient can take.'

'How can he tell how much bad news a patient is ready for when he barely knows her?'

I sighed and Emma looked at me.

'There's nothing worse than waiting for results. You feel stuck in limbo, don't you? Do you remember what William and I did the weekend before my prognosis? We drove to Harlech and went up to the top of Snowdon on the train. I remember looking down from the summit and thinking that whatever happened to me in the future, nothing would be that important – not compared with the beauty of that view from the mountain.'

Emma moved over to the kitchen window and stared out at the closely packed houses opposite and the narrow strip of white sky above them.

'The feeling wore off a bit when I got home, but I still remember it.'

She took a photograph out of her handbag and passed it to me. 'That was one of the best days of my life', she said.

The photo showed her alone, cheeks wet with rain, pale curls flying in the wind, looking out across a deep valley to a magnificent grey-green ridge.

My oncologist's face was impassive, giving no hint of his knowledge of my prognosis and the future intent of my biological cells. He shook my hand and waved me to the seat next to his desk. Paul sat down next to me.

I tried to remain calm. I focused on the wise advice given to Stephen Russell's Urban Warrior in my favourite book of the moment. The advice was to maintain a calm view of the world and your place in it, whatever is happening, and not to take yourself too seriously: 'don't get overexcited or panicked.'

The wisdom of this was obvious. Yes, it's better to face whatever happens from a stable state of equilibrium. Because I identified with this philosophy so strongly, I knew that I could take whatever Dr Shah told me, good or bad, in my stride.

Despite this confidence, I found myself sitting rigidly upright as if my body was a hard sheet of plastic, just like the chair I was sitting on.

The oncologist spoke deliberately.

'Your cancer was found to be grade 1.'

He paused, unaware of the fact that my heart was jolting in my chest.

'Your cancer was sensitive to the female sex hormone, oestrogen.'

I was trying to breathe without panting.

The oncologist looked at me and then carried on.

'This is good news because it means that hormonal treatment will be able to block the hormones that encourage a cancer to grow.'

He slowly listed other aspects of my cancer – the nuclear grade, the formation of the cells. My eyes were fixed on his angular face and I was waiting, waiting for the words that I wanted to hear – and this time, they came.

'We removed eight lymph nodes and they were all clear.'

These words propelled me into elation mode. It was as if I had never heard of the Urban Warrior, never recognised Jane Kenyon's cautionary image of the 'drunken monkey.' My whole body seemed to liquefy with the torrent of relief coursing through it.

I trembled. 'Oh ... that's great.'

While this was going on, Paul was becoming disconcerted. In a medical setting, hospital or surgery, he was inured to the emotionally distanced, objective role of scientific doctor, and he couldn't ease himself out of it.

'She's been reading all about it on the Internet', he explained to the consultant.

The oncologist was too used to giving bad news to pass up the joy of the occasion.

'It's good news', he said. 'You'll be given a course of radiotherapy but you won't need chemotherapy.' He smiled at me.

A further rush of emotion came over me. This time it was directed towards the oncologist himself, the person who recognised and respected my euphoria, and it felt like love. It was the counterpoint to the dislike I had felt for my surgeon on that sunny day when he'd told me that my lump was cancerous.

'Thank you so much', I said.

I hesitated and then the words poured out: 'You're the nicest person I've ever met.'

I shook his large hand with its long sensitive fingers and felt as if I was forever bonded with him, this wonderful wise man who had set me free from worry.

Once I was outside in the corridor again, I looked at the other patients who were still waiting for examination, diagnosis or prognosis. I pitied them. I had been set free. I had nothing more to worry about. My life could carry on as normal.

Back home, we pulled into our drive just as my nextdoor neighbour, Mary, and her sister were getting out of their car on the other side of the holly hedge that separated us. I hurried round it.

'There was no cancer in any of my lymph nodes. It's a really good sign. I'm just so relieved.'

They didn't understand what I was excited about, but they had known the lead-up to the verdict and were happy to go along with my relief. They gave me congratulatory smiles.

'We're absolutely delighted for you.'

Within the next year, Mary was to be diagnosed with breast cancer and four lymph nodes were found to be cancerous. I just hoped she had forgotten this scene because by then I was embarrassed by its triumphalism. No doubt the author of my Urban Warrior book was thinking of scenarios like this, as well as the personal implications, when he advised cool composure in the face of triumph as well as disaster.

Throughout that evening the phone kept ringing with friends checking on my results. I treated them all to the same upbeat report. My lymph nodes were clear. I would be having radiotherapy but no chemotherapy. I had nothing more to worry about.

When I awoke the next morning, the previous day's good news came rushing into my mind. Yesterday's euphoria had faded, but not into a realistic acceptance of the nature of my disease. Instead it seemed to me that it was only feasible that the lymph nodes should have been clear and that I was now clear of cancer. It fitted in with the story of my life to date. Things usually turned out fairly well for me when it came to health matters. Why had I ever had any doubts about it? I was one of nature's naturally healthy people, like my mother and my grandmothers. I had little to fear from cancer. The threat was over and, apart from my paralysed arm and the radiotherapy still to come, I was on my way back to normal.

That afternoon we attended our local grey-stone church for the wedding of the son of close friends. Listening to the familiar service and surrounded by old friends, I began to feel part of normal life again. We had all watched the bridegroom grow up from an impish lad to become a professional artist. We had shared milestones like anniversaries and weddings over the years, and my identity in the group was reassuringly fixed and unchanging.

Coming out of the church after the ceremony, I was shocked to find that many friends greeted me as if I were not my normal self but still a patient.

'How are you?'

'How's your arm?'

'When do you start your radiotherapy?'

Each time someone spoke I reacted as if I was on trial and my life depended on convincing them that I was not going to die. Far from it – I was a super-patient and super-lucky and therefore back to my normal self.

'I've got a very good prognosis ... I've been lucky. My lymph nodes were clear.'

My arm was still paralysed, but the rest of my body had been exonerated by the oncologist. I was a normal person again, not a fully fledged patient.

On that wedding day I was feeling the compulsion to maintain appearances that had been drilled into me since childhood. I should strive to retain my persona as a capable person, otherwise others would reject me – so I carried on talking up my prognosis.

As we walked away from the church past the lichen-covered gravestones, it occurred to me that although I was assuring others that my prognosis was good, I had not asked the oncologist – the cancer expert – to give me his opinion. He had told me the results of the tests, but I hadn't followed up by asking him directly what my prognosis was. It hadn't even occurred to me to ask him.

I began to long to talk to other women who shared my fears and who might even have spent time whistling in the dark just as I was doing, and my thoughts turned to Emma's support group, Bosom Friends. Each of its members would, like me and like Jane Kenyon's unknown figure in the woods, have 'walked alone in the chill of the dawn' and might also have seen the grey shape of an owl fly overhead.

CHAPTER 12

Soul sisters

'You'll get stuck', Julie, friend and arch-sceptic, warned me when she saw my Bosom Friends newsletter lying on the coffee table. On its cover page was a photograph of a group of women in slinky evening dresses, arms linked and smiling into the camera.

Julie pointed a finger, 'Like them.'

She flicked her long brown hair back from her face and trained her fierce glance on me. 'If you join Bosom Friends, you'll just be mixing with other cancer patients instead of moving on with your life. I know what happens. You sign on, and then in no time at all it becomes your whole life.'

'It's just a support group', I said. 'Not a cult.'

'I'd stay away if I were you. You need to get on with real life and forget about your illness whenever you can.'

It was the evening of my first visit to Bosom Friends, the support group that had given me a unique kind of help when I was in hospital. The 'Helpline' poster in the hospital corridor while I waited to hear my diagnosis, the scarlet and green floral bag for toting my drain around, and the bedside visit from Ruth, the committee member, had all signified that others were out there thinking of me, other women who lived in the same world and had made the same journey as me. Now I was going to meet those other women in person.

Since leaving hospital I had felt as if I were in no man's land, but the group members might be able to give me hints about who I now was, what I should do next, and how I should go about finding the best way to live. I would be able to look at them and the way that they lived their lives and, with their help, work out the dos and don'ts of living through serious illness.

Gaia had told me that a support group like Bosom Friends was a gathering of people with the same illness or condition who meet to share information, experiences, problems and solutions. At a support group patients can express their fears and frustrations safe in the knowledge that other members are going through what they are going through and can understand their thoughts and feelings. Some research results claim that patients who attend support groups improve their self-esteem and even their health outcomes, whether for cancer, arthritis, spinal injuries, tinnitus or any other illness or disability. All in all it seemed like a good idea, even an obligation, that anyone who wants to be a good patient should attend a support group.

Yet I still felt nervous. The truth was that Julie had voiced some of the fears that I had been trying hard to suppress. I was fearful about going to

Bosom Friends because I was not sure exactly what it entailed. Julie might turn out to be right – I might get stuck in the role of patient long after I should have moved back to my normal life. After all, my disease had only affected my body – there was no reason why my mind should become involved. I might become dependent on the group emotionally, which would make it difficult to resume my old state of mind ... blah, blah, blah. I was getting bogged down. As the Barefoot Doctor in my copy of Russell's *Barefoot Doctor's Handbook for the Urban Warrior* said, 'Worrying is nothing more than a conditioned, knee-jerk, reflexive reaction.' The good patient doesn't get twittery but takes action.

There were many reasons why I felt that I should go to Bosom Friends, and not just the ones that Gaia had mentioned. I needed to get some kind of life outside my home, but at the same time I still felt like a patient, dependent on the hospital staff and too fragile to face the outside world. Bosom Friends was a halfway house, not medical but not non-medical either – the perfect compromise.

Emma was already a member and she was convinced that I would benefit in the same way that she had from belonging to the group. She drove me to the meeting which was held regularly in the Postgraduate Centre, a squat building inside the Parkside Hospital grounds. I was back on the territory that had become so familiar to me, and where I felt I still belonged. The Centre was next to the towering six-floor hospital wing that I had left only a few weeks before and, walking from the car park, I looked up wistfully at the window of the fourth-floor room that had been mine. Fear and sadness made up many of my memories, but it was the good memories that shocked me. The time I had spent in hospital that I had dreaded so much before I went in had turned out to be not only absorbing but even sometimes enjoyable. Everything I had experienced in that room was in technicolour in my memory – a time of fear and sorrow but also of drama, of feelings of connection with others, and a feeling of being stretched, of learning new facts and ideas. I stored away this surprising new take on my hospital incarceration to think about at some other time.

A small group of women stood talking in the vestibule, and when they saw Emma they called her over and began to ask her questions about the extent of her hair loss during her chemotherapy.

As I hovered on the edge of the group, I noticed two women coming through the entrance. One of them was wearing a familiar red and blue velvet hairband. It was Samira Khan, the woman whom I'd met at Rushwood Hospital just two days after finding my suspicious lump. She came over to ask how I was.

After a while she said quietly 'Do you remember what I said about having cancer when I saw you at the hospital?'

'Yes, I've been thinking about that.'

'Well, I've had another mastectomy since then ... but ... I still feel the same way ...'.

Her friend broke in and ushered her away to sign into the meeting. 'See you later', Samira said.

A woman with spiky red hair approached me. 'Hi, I'm Sheryl. Are you a new member?'

'Yes, I came out of hospital a couple of weeks ago so I'm still adapting. Everything seems a bit strange and unreal.'

'Excuse me scratching my head. This wig's new and it's a bit itchy.' She rubbed her fingers into the nape of her neck. 'Yes, I know exactly what you mean. It's a long haul back to feeling normal, and I suppose you've still got the chemo to go through?'

'No, not chemo, but I'll be starting radiotherapy at some stage.'

It seemed to me that I had been through only part of the usual group initiation procedure. I hadn't shared the bonding experience of chemotherapy and the group counselling sessions that followed it. I could hear the women beside me talking about these experiences. Some of them had sat in the same room together while the drugs seeped into their bloodstream. They knew what regimes the others were following, how long each session lasted and what drugs they were on, depending on the stage of cancer and the type of cancer cell. I had been spared the ordeal of chemotherapy, but might one or two of the other women think that my kind of cancer was less valid than theirs?

'Has everyone here had chemotherapy?' I asked Sheryl, looking at the other women.

'We've got women who've had every type of treatment here. There are women who've had a lumpectomy and no further treatment, women who've had chemo and no radio, and women like me who are on a second or third course of chemo.'

She smiled at me. 'I know what you're worried about. Everyone's nervous when they first come. They're not sure how they're going to fit in.'

'Yes, I feel a bit like that', I said.

'I know. I felt the same way. I know you'll get something out of coming here. Everybody's experience is valued. There are all kinds of breast cancer, and it's frightening whatever sort of treatment you have to go through.'

I sat down at the end of a row of seats and glanced at the sheets of paper I had found on my chair. They turned out to be the latest newsletter and the minutes of the last meeting.

'What are *you* doing here, may I ask?'

The woman seated in the row in front had turned around to face me. It was Laura, a fellow student on the website design course that we'd completed three months previously. In the pub after the lessons we had talked about all kinds of subjects, but she'd never mentioned breast cancer.

'I'm here because I had a breast cancer op a few weeks ago', I said. 'How about you?'

'Fifteen years ago. I had the works – mastectomy, chemo, radio. And no problems since.'

'That's good to hear.'

'Yes, I like to come here every so often and tell people about it. They find it reassuring. I'm proof that breast cancer isn't a death sentence.'

Later that evening I met a former colleague, a neighbour and one of the staff at my local library. These women, like Laura, belonged to my 'normal life', but now it turned out that they also belonged in my 'illness life.' The realisation dawned that any group of women over the age of forty is likely to include a small number of women who have been treated for breast cancer.

Why had the women I knew already never mentioned their illness to me?

Laura told me, 'I rarely speak about my cancer now. Not outside of here anyway. You find that sometimes people get embarrassed and then you wish you'd never mentioned it.'

I remembered the day after my diagnosis when I had longed to tell the unknowing Nicholas of Middleton Hall about my cancer, despite the fact that it would have been embarrassingly inappropriate. That had been my first exercise in keeping my disease under wraps.

'That's why women like coming to Bosom Friends', Laura said. 'Cancer's just ordinary here and you can relax.'

Yes, ordinary. I had once found it easy to imagine myself as a special person, unusually struck down by a devastating disease, even a kind of a heroine. I still did sometimes. But there was a new kind of freedom in recognising the falsity of this perception and the depressing way in which it disconnects you from others.

As Emma had once told me months ago, when as far as I was concerned 'Bosom Friends' was just a sentimental-sounding name, '*I feel normal when I'm at Bosom Friends.*'

It was only now that I was beginning to understand what she meant. First, I was among other women patients so I could relax. There was no need to make those tiny micro-decisions about how I, a lone patient, was going to present my illness to a healthy listener. Secondly, I had listened to the medics and their medical terms and tried to become familiar with their language of disease, but now it was a relief to be in a community where the patient's own personal experience of her illness was the focus of conversation, not the biological facts about her disease.

I became entranced by the way that the women told their stories and encouraged me to tell mine. The warm harmonics of shared experience but richly individual stories contrasted with the lopsided dialogues of hospital consultations. 'Stories', said the poet, Ted Hughes, 'are hospitals where we heal, where our imaginations are healed.' As I listened to how others spoke about their bodies, I reinterpreted my own experiences. The altered parts of my body – my scar, my missing lymph nodes, my limp arm and hand – yes, they were all part of my being. They legitimately played a role in my life and weren't just hidden extras to the facts considered important by the professionals.

Laura told me that the support group had been going for eight years. It had been founded by Carys, the charismatic consultant nurse who was now working in a London teaching hospital, who had helped me so much in the early days of my treatment. It had grown in numbers and importance over the years and acquired influence both in the hospital and outside in the community.

'If you look at the statement of accounts attached to the minutes of the last meeting, you can see that we handle a large budget', Laura said. 'There's stuff in the newsletter if you want to know about what we do to help.'

The newsletter listed the support group's main priorities – to provide emotional support to patients diagnosed with breast cancer, to raise awareness in the local community so that people would seek diagnosis and treatment at an early stage, and to raise funds to provide practical support where it was needed, such as help with visits to hospital and folding wheelchairs.

The newsletter explained that Carys's vision when she founded the group was to connect women with breast cancer with each other for support and friendship, and also to make connections with the medical staff. Into my mind came the memory of E M Forster's novel, *Howards End*, and its mantra 'Only connect.' Through her work with patients and hospital staff, Carys had learned how difficult it is to make the connections that she realised were so important.

As I was reading the newsletter, Sheryl arrived at my side with a small, energetic woman in tow.

'This is Nicky', Sheryl said. 'She's the chairman and I'm a member of her committee – one of her slaves.' She patted Nicky on the shoulder, messing up the neat folds of her blue silk scarf.

'One of fifteen wonderful ladies', Nicky said, readjusting the drape of the scarf across her shoulders. 'There's no limit to the number on the committee, and any woman who wants to join us is welcomed with open arms.'

She stepped on to the stage and introduced herself to the gathering. She asked any new members to raise their hands, and then appeared to look straight at me. I uncertainly raised my left hand. A couple of other women also raised their hands, and the other members looked round at us, nodding and smiling in welcome.

The talk was about reconstruction, and was given by a plastic surgeon who listed the many advantages of breast 'reconstruction' – a persuasive word which implies that all will be renewed as it was before. I remembered my own confused feelings about it when I was trying to make a rational choice between mastectomy and lumpectomy. Now it almost seemed as if a reconstruction operation was in itself conducive to regaining health.

The surgeon's enthusiasm alienated some of the women sitting around me. They started muttering among themselves:

'I'm happy as I am ...'

'I don't need another op ...'

The surgeon seemed unaware of the diversity of the views, values and experiences of his audience. Some were contemplating reconstruction; some had already had the operation, some were against it because they didn't want to go through another operation, and others thought it was unnecessary.

When the surgeon asked whether anyone had any questions, a woman wearing a purple and pink striped hat put up her hand.

'I'm happy as I am. I don't want a reconstruction. Have you got anything to say to people like me?'

The surgeon paused.

'I wouldn't want to encourage anyone to go ahead with reconstruction who wasn't 100% sure that she wanted it', he said. 'It's a big operation, and I hope I haven't been giving the impression that it's an easy decision. As a plastic surgeon I explain the pros and cons, but I'm used to speaking to women who have already decided on it. I personally think it's a wonderful operation, but it's not for everyone, and many, many women are happy without it.'

The original speaker nodded and smiled at him. 'Thank you. I agree with that completely.'

I was to find that the surgeon's indirect admission that his talk had been one-sided was just one of a number of occasions when doctors visiting as speakers seemed to reflect and learn from the women at Bosom Friends, as well as the other way around.

Carys's original vision for the support group had reminded me of the mantra in *Howards End,* 'only connect.' Another of Forster's novels, *A Passage to India,* also came into my mind at this meeting. The previous year I had analysed the novel with some of my students, and one of them had half-jokingly pointed out its relevance to the partition between lecturers and students.

The novel portrays the English and the Indians in colonial India. They stare at each other across a cultural divide and a history of imbalanced power relations and mutual suspicion, and Forster wonders whether connection is even possible. His conclusion is that it can be achieved not by political campaigning, but by individual social connections.

Bosom Friends was an organisation that enabled the kind of détente that Foster envisaged. Patients and medical staff met on territory that was convenient and familiar to both groups, and the meetings were times when attitudes sometimes shifted and when some of the traditional barriers between medical experts and patients were lifted.

At the meeting with the plastic surgeon, there was no speaker to give reasons for not having a reconstruction to balance his recommendations, and it was only the question from the woman in the striped hat that had made the treatment of the subject more even-handed. Support groups have no mandate to ensure that issues are presented in a balanced way, but I was to find that the informal discussions after the talks usually went some way towards restoring the balance.

After the plastic surgeon had left, we gathered in the small lobby next to the lecture room for a tea break. Lack of space forced us into an intermingling group instead of the twosomes and individuals who had sat scattered in the large lecture hall.

One woman revealed that her reconstruction involved moving fat up from her abdomen to her chest wall, and she had been surprised and appalled at the amount of pain involved.

Another had been disappointed to find that the reconstructed breasts were as big and saggy as her original ones.

'I told the consultant that I'd expected that he would give me smaller, perkier breasts.'

He told me, 'Well, you didn't say anything beforehand.'

'I was thrilled with my op', one woman said. 'It gave me back my confidence so I could start getting back to normal.'

There was talk about the discomfort of wigs, the difficulties of dealing with the emotions and expectations of relatives, and the effects of chemotherapy.

I had learned a lot from the plastic surgeon's talk but now, unofficially, I was learning much more.

Some of the women were wearing the little pink ribbon bows that raised so much money for breast cancer charities. Soon after my diagnosis I had been given a large envelope, in exactly the same shade of pink, containing a sheaf of leaflets and booklets. I had stared with distaste at the colour – that infantilising 'baby pink.' Do women with breast cancer have no choice? Is it a case of 'get breast cancer, get branded with pinkness'?

But after that first visit to Bosom Friends, other associations began to kick in. The pink newsletter giving information about sources of help, dates of outings and charity events. Pictures in the lobby of members wearing pink wigs and doing a fundraising moonlit walk in London. There was a snapshot of Emma, wearing the pink logo ribbon on the occasion when she had been awarded membership of the city's society of artists. She had been determined to wear the ribbon on all occasions in a bid to raise awareness of breast cancer, but as an artist she had been wryly amused by the way that the pastel pink clashed with her red waistcoat and red patterned shirt.

There's a whole world out there related to cancer, I realised. There are public research institutions and huge charities dedicated to giving information or raising funds for research, and there are activists campaigning for better access to healthcare and better research into the links between cancer and the environment. Cancer doesn't exist in a medical vacuum, but has public significance over and above its biology.

Thanks to Bosom Friends, issues like prioritising, funding and the role of corporate charity began to have personal meaning for me even during those early days when I was still inwardly focused. The activists in the support group had become open to what Audre Lorde refers to as 'the need for every woman to live a considered life.' In doing so, women become less willing 'to passively accept external and destructive controls over our lives and our identities.' There were many different kinds of significance hanging around ready to attach themselves to our sickness. Cancer was linked to the outside world in more ways – political, social, economic, and so on – than I had ever imagined. Being ill was not a singular event that happened to the individual in isolation.

The Bosom Friends newsletter had a list of forthcoming guest speakers, some of them from the beauty industry. Over the coming months I was to find that these speakers were dedicated to maintaining our 'femininity.' They included local beauticians, lingerie saleswomen and wigmakers. In contrast with the approach of Nicky the chairman and the committee, who were grounded in shared knowledge and experience, the guest speakers sometimes revealed a hint of pressure even though their talks were full of the fun of fashion and make-up:

'Your appearance is one of the most important things about you, as a woman, and you must keep yourself looking attractive even though you've got breast cancer.'

'About to lose your hair? There are some lovely wigs.'

'Having chemo and losing your eyelashes? You can use false ones instead.'

Some women welcomed this advice, some were indifferent, and other rejected it, making remarks like:

'Who wants to bother with false eyelashes? People can take me or leave me.'

Voices like these were never heard on the floor to balance up the range of options, because the group depended on people with commercial interests to come and give unpaid talks, and in any case their talks were genuinely interesting and often helpful.

So many women, so many opinions and so many feelings – overlapping, merging and diverging. I became aware of two creeds, each of them caricatures, but between them covering the polarities of values and beliefs among the members, especially when it came to being a good patient. They reflected the continuum of thoughts of any one individual, myself included:

Creed A

I am a good patient.
I do what the doctors and nurses tell me.
I have a positive attitude that will help me to beat my cancer.
I keep myself looking good by taking care with my make-up, hair and clothes.

I try to keep myself slim.

If my hair falls out, I will wear a wig, however itchy or uncomfortable it is.

If my eyelashes fall out, I will go to the beauty salon to learn how to apply false ones.

I will work hard to find the right kind of prosthesis and bra.

Chemotherapy and radiotherapy make me tired, but I rarely complain.

Cancer has made me realise my own mortality, so I will be much nicer to everyone in future.

I worry about my partner's reaction to my illness, because my damaged body might alter his estimation of me.

Whatever happens to me, I will behave in an uncomplaining, devoted and selfless way towards my partner/children/family/friends.

I aim to get over this as soon as possible.

Creed B

I am a good patient.

I am entitled to help and support.

I will assess any help that I am offered to make sure that it suits my needs.

I will help other women with breast cancer and show them that it is not so bad – you can still be a real flawed person, you don't have to be a saint.

The threat of mortality has made me realise that I have a right to a life of my own choosing.

I am able to grumble and change my mind and my moods at this difficult time.

I am free to accept or reject all the reconstruction/prosthesis stuff and still be attractive and normal.

I am learning and growing as a result of my illness experiences.

There was no one woman who embodied either of these extremes, but these two creeds hung in the air over every conversation, gradually giving us the opportunity to recognise the individuality and the contradictory nature of our reactions and feelings, and to absorb the idea that there are a myriad of ways to respond to the challenges of illness and its treatment, not just one.

My mission to be a good patient was becoming more difficult and at the same time more easy because it was becoming apparent to me that there was not just one 'good patient identity', not just one integral way of being and one way of acting that mark out the good patient, but countless ways.

Maybe there was no Holy Grail, no magic formula, to strive for at the end of my treatment, just constant attempts to do the best one can. I began to wonder whether striving to return to my old, pre-illness life was fruit-less. Perhaps I should be like so many of the women at Bosom Friends and strive to embrace the challenges thrown up by illness, and even welcome the changes that they brought.

The group was helping me to realise that the challenges I faced were not peculiar to me. And it was helping me to move my focus outwards to others and the outside world. Paradoxically, it was the group's minority status in the community that was a help and a strength in doing this.

Since my diagnosis, I had sometimes felt patronised as a member of a minority group – 'patient with life-threatening illness.'

'People eat far too much junk food these days – chips and beefburgers and so on. That's the cause of all these cancers ... though not yours, I'm sure', said an acquaintance.

'Live in the moment – that's what you've got to do, isn't it?' said a well-intentioned colleague as he stopped to exchange a few casual words with me in our local off-licence. The philosophy that he was referring to was suddenly reduced to a simple and natty technique to distract the marginalised and afflicted from mortal thoughts.

Remarks like these were clumsy but benevolent attempts to reassure someone who the speaker viewed as 'other.' They were similar to remarks relating to my Welsh origins, such as the reassurance that I could almost pass for normal: 'You haven't got that much of a Welsh accent.'

It was only when I first left Wales in my early twenties and became a Welsh exile in an English community that I fully appreciated my cultural identity and hence my links with other minority cultures. As a member of Bosom Friends, a group that was a part of and at the same time outside our local community, there was a re-run of the same lesson – that vulnerability is a kind of strength and a bond. Living on the edge can spark off self-knowledge. Membership of a minority group can nurture feelings of connection with others, whatever their affiliation.

It was at a Bosom Friends meeting that I first came across the overt mention of death in relation to my disease. When it comes to sensitive subjects, support groups have to consider the feelings of people who have diverse experiences of illness and come from different environments. Dying was something that Bosom Friends might have wanted to avoid acknowledging. After all, there was an inevitable, ongoing trickle of deaths among support group members. They could have been forgiven for taking the safer option of silence, but they were braver than that. I was shocked at that first meeting when they announced the recent death of a member. Surely in the circumstances it would be better to keep upbeat and not frighten new members. Nicky talked briefly about Madeline, her love for her two young sons, her jokes and her zest for partying. Other members contributed their fond anecdotes. 'We will always remember Madeline, dancing', Nicky concluded. There were murmurs of assent. The sadness and joy of facing the challenges of cancer seemed to mingle in the room.

Newcomers like me absorbed this light and shade and were able to glimpse the fact that here was a world in which it was possible that not just our hopes, but even our bleakest thoughts and fears might be shared by others.

Later that week I heard two cancer 'survivors', both minor novelists, being interviewed on a national radio programme. They voiced the kind of opinions that reminded me of my friend Julie and her warning words about Bosom Friends and 'getting stuck.'

They referred to women who 'make a little career out of cancer.' They agreed that this was the way in which these unfortunate women compensated for lives that were not working out. Better to 'get back to the real world', to 'get on with your life', just as they had. The writers described the very same fears that I had experienced before my first visit to Bosom Friends – that I might get stuck and dependent or life might pass me by while I was involved with a marginal group. Now I knew better. Bosom Friends, with its mission for connection and its practical support in the face of distress and disruption, was itself the real world, in all its grittiness.

CHAPTER 13

Side-effects

I wanted to be like Emma – the kind of patient who inspires other women or at the very least doesn't dishearten them, the kind that passes through each stage of her treatment not necessarily smoothly, but steadily and valiantly. Yet eight weeks after my operation, with another four weeks to wait before I started my radiotherapy treatment, my body felt alien and I was overcome with self-pity. How much of this was due to my illness and how much was due to my disablement? My arm and hand were still paralysed. I had what the medics call 'finger drop' as well as 'wrist drop.'

Having entered hospital with my road mapped out before me – operation, post-operation convalescence, radiotherapy, recovery – I had now fallen by the wayside, unsure of what to do next and filled with the sense of disruption that Brody identifies in his book, *Stories of Sickness*:

> If sickness leads us to see our bodies as being something foreign, thwarting our wills by their intransigence and unmanageability, then sickness has fundamentally altered our experience of self and has introduced a sense of split and disruption where formerly unity reigned.

In just a few short months my body had rebelled against and rejected its lowly place in my mind. Now it was at the forefront of my thinking. For better or worse, I would never regain my former casual faith in my body and its efficacy. I envied others who were still able to think of their bodies and minds, their thoughts and actions, as integral. My paralysed hand was the graphic representation of my feelings of disruption, and for a time I became obsessed by the contrast between my own useless, floppy hand and the clever, animated hands of others.

One Saturday afternoon during the long wait before I started my radiotherapy, I went with Paul to a party given by our friend Julie and her partner, Roger. After everyone had eaten, I stood watching Emma as she collected the empty plates, her right hand picking up each plate between fingers and thumb and placing it on a pile that she balanced against her body and supported with her outstretched left hand.

Julie asked her how she was.

'I'm fine thanks, Julie. Fairly well recovered.' She flicked some straggling curls back off her face with the curved fingers of her right hand. 'I've even stopped looking at other women's bosoms now. For the first few weeks after my mastectomy I couldn't stop staring at breasts.'

She laughed at the look of surprise on Julie's face.

'Jealousy, I suppose. I'd lost one of mine ... so my mind just got stuck on breasts.'

Emma cast a glance at me as I stood watching them.

I realised that I had been staring at their hands, my eyes moving from Emma's hands to Julie's and back again. I had become obsessed with other people's hands and their miraculous complexity in the same kind of way that Emma had briefly become obsessed with breasts. I found myself comparing the loss of the use of an arm with the loss of a breast, just as if there was a hierarchy of suffering.

Many women associate the shock of breast cancer with the loss of a breast and its attendant worries. There is the loss of the old familiar landscape of the body, the bewildering change in the distribution of weight, the discomfort of a prosthesis, and often the pain and stress of a reconstruction. Then there are the fears of loss of femininity and of others' reactions to the loss of one's breast in a society where physical appearance is so important.

How does this kind of loss compare with losing the use of a functionally vital part of the body, such as a limb? Although my disablement limited my activities, my arm and hand were still there – no surgeon's knife had sliced them off and thrown them into a surgical waste bin. My paralysis was the result of a mechanical failure, a crushed nerve which would probably regenerate in time.

When I consulted Gaia, my Internet muse, I discovered that there are 27 bones, 33 muscles and 20 joints in each hand. How amazing to think that they were all still there in my right hand, none of them of any use but just lying there, dormant. No wonder I focused on the constantly moving hands of family and friends.

When visitors came, it was sometimes difficult to concentrate on what they were saying because their hands magnetised my eyes. They rarely kept them still. When a hand was not moving or handling an object, it would be scratching or massaging its partner or stroking the chin or brushing hair back off the face. Some visitors used their hands to emphasise their points – quick, slow, large or small movements of the hands and arms according to their personalities and the mood of their speech. They seemed oblivious of their gestures.

I had once been like them, unaware of my gestures except for those captured mid-speech on camera. Now, with one arm silent at my side, I felt as if my speech was muffled.

Watching Meg dicing some carrots, her left hand steadying the carrot between thumb and fingers, and her right hand slashing quickly and rhythmically with a sharp knife, it was difficult to believe that I had once been able to use my hands precisely, just like that. And it was difficult to believe that I had once been the nurturant mother, the sole provider of meals for the family. Now I was just a spectator – a sidelined mother.

Gaia had told me that all tools and engines on earth are only extensions of human limbs and senses. One of the features that distinguish us humans from all other animals is the way that we can use our thumbs. Chimpanzees, gorillas and several other creatures have thumbs, but only the human thumb can rotate about its base and can touch and be put in direct opposition to each finger. This means that we can grasp objects of varying shapes and sizes, manipulate them and perform delicate operations. This, combined with the ability to reason and make choices, led us to invent tools.

My paralysed right hand was unable to grip any of these tools, but I could use many of them one-handed so long as I took my time over each operation. The toaster, blender and kettle all helped me to prepare food and drink with only my left hand. The washing machine and tumble dryer enabled me to deal with the laundry. Before my illness I had used these tools and pieces of equipment daily, but only now did I feel surprised gratitude towards the inventors who had enabled so many people like me to be independent as a result of their inventions.

Even playing the piano one-handed was easier thanks to the invention of a musical tool – the sustaining pedal – way back in the eighteenth century. The pedal made it possible to let one or more tones keep on sounding after the keys had been released. Striking other keys immediately afterwards gave the illusion that I was actually playing in several places on the keyboard at the same time, just as if I had two working hands.

Since my return from hospital, I had been practising 'Left's Turn Only', a boogie piece for one hand composed by Robert Vandall. It had been a happy surprise to come across such a pertinent piece among my piles of sheet music. Through Gaia I learned that it was but one of a surprisingly large repertoire of piano music for the left hand alone. Some of it had been specifically written for disabled pianists like Paul Wittgenstein, who lost his right arm in the First World War. Given this existing body of music specifically written for others who shared my plight, there was no escaping the fact that life is full of contingencies. How naive my former wonder at my unusual side-effect – my paralysed right arm and hand – had been. Now playing the boogie piece linked me to others who also loved music, loved playing the piano, had lost the use of their right hand and had moved on to playing the piano one-handed.

Losing the use of my arm had altered my conception of myself and my relationship with the world in an even more intrinsic way than my breast cancer diagnosis. It had made me reconsider every action and every plan, and made me realise that aspects of myself which I had thought were fundamental were not really so after all. I wasn't naturally good at running a house with all of its chores like ironing, cooking and shopping, or at playing the piano. These activities and many others were contingent on my having two working hands. My hybrid identity as a mother, writer, lecturer, pianist and so on had been shown to be precarious and fluid, not magically fixed and integral to myself as a person as I had assumed. All of these identities were merged with my capacity to use my right arm and hand as capably as I used my left arm and hand.

Many weeks previously, I had viewed my life as well ordered and progressive, but now here I was with a disease and a paralysed arm. Life could switch so quickly. I was haunted by the thoughts of a woman who had suffered a much more horrible catastrophe than mine. Her face and hands had been badly burned in a terrible rail crash a few years previously when a fireball had engulfed the carriage in which she was sitting. She was in hospital for more than three months, and had undergone several major operations to graft skin from her inner arms and thighs on to her hands.

I had read about her suffering long before my own operation, and had felt horrified by the pain and misery that she must be feeling. I had empathised with her. I had understood her feelings by imagining myself in her situation, and thoughts of her suffering had haunted me long afterwards.

When I had awoken the morning after my operation and found my arm and hand still paralysed, I had thought of her, as I had when I slid slowly out of bed and tried to carry on normal everyday activities like washing and eating.

My fear, helplessness and other emotions had given me a new insight into the reality of her experience, highlighting the hopeless limitations of my pre-operation 'empathy' and the fact that empathy is limited by one's own experience.

This realisation turned the world into a more complex and threatening one than I had ever understood before my operation. My underestimation of the range and depth of suffering of the woman in the rail crash was an indication of my failure on a more global scale. Whether in relation to famine, genocide or civil war, I now knew that I could no longer count on my 'empathy' to comprehend the full extent of the suffering of the individuals involved and the horrific disruption of their lives.

This realisation haunted me in yet another way during this time of introspection. Violent criminals, so psychologists tell us, often lack empathy due to having had abusive childhoods. This doesn't exonerate them, but lack of adult care and compassion would certainly have stunted their capacity for empathy. Now I was closer to those criminals than I'd thought, because I had recognised my own limitations with regard to empathy. The difference between myself and the criminals was not absolute, but one of degree.

This insight was a more negative but strangely parallel version of my vision in the garden centre. There I had been inspired by feeling part of a spiritual and timeless common humanity. Now I recognised the empathy shortfalls that linked me with society's outsiders and that made them less 'outside' and less remote from me than I had previously imagined. Illness was at one and the same time extending and revealing the limits of my imagination.

After the New York City twin towers disaster of September 11, 2001, novelist Ian McEwan commented that 'Imagining what it is like to be someone other than yourself is at the core of our humanity. It is the essence of compassion, and it is the beginning of morality.'

Empathy is an action, not a result. Empathy is not a conjuring act that replicates the other's experience within one's own mind and emotions, and if we could have perfect empathy towards everyone at once, we would be overwhelmed and paralysed by all the suffering in the world. But as David Hume, the eighteenth-century philosopher, points out, having a reasonable degree of empathy at least for those immediately around us saves people from selfishness and barbarity. The process may prove to be imperfect – my imagination had failed to envisage the full extent of the rail crash survivor's anguish – but the mere act of opening oneself to the experience of the other person is enough. As McEwan implies, it is in the actual act of imagining that enlightenment lies.

As I began to tell my story to the consultant neurologist, my voice took on a whiny tone. An ordinary everyday operation had resulted in what was a catastrophe for me, and although my rational mind was forgiving, I still felt some free-floating anger about it.

'I came to after the operation and found that my arm and hand were dead, completely paralysed.'

At the end of my account, I made an attempt at a joke: 'I think I'll have to sue the operating staff.'

At the word 'sue', the consultant folded his arms and surveyed me with steely eyes and pursed lips. He was one of them. He identified not with me but with other doctors, particularly my surgeon and my anaesthetist.

He explained that he was going to find out which nerves were affected. He placed electrodes on my hands and administered a series of small shocks. The tests confirmed that my radial nerve was crushed – radial nerve dysfunction or 'radial neuropathy' as the consultant called it. He told me that although he had seen only one other patient with this problem, he was optimistic.

'The most likely prognosis is complete restoration and recovery', he said.

It was as if he was promising me a return to my former self, and I was excited, forgetting all about the women at Bosom Friends and my admiration for the way in which they had embraced the changes that illness brought. The consultant's words were an omen that I would return unchanged to my pre-illness life. The gods were on my side.

Charmaine, a friend who works as an arts administrator, rang the next morning. 'I've got a proposition that I think would be good for you. There's a group called "Mirage" – they work for Music in the Community. Their keyboard player is ill and I thought of you. Would you fancy performing with them at a concert at a residential home for elderly people?'

'How can I do that with one hand?'

'I heard you improvising all those pieces one-handed when I came over last week. This will be a piece of cake. You'll know all the songs they're singing – they're all well-known ones. Just improvise with your left hand, like you've been doing. Give them some arpeggios and a bit of the tune.'

I hesitated.

'Don't worry. You can do it. I'll tell them that your right arm is paralysed, but I won't tell them anything else', Charmaine said.

As Jaz, the group's compère, drove us over to the old people's home, I was reminded of my meeting with Nicholas at Middleton Hall the day after my diagnosis. Once again I was with strangers who knew nothing of my illness, and once again I was aware of how deeply I was immersed in the world of illness. The difference was that this time it felt liberating to be in the outside world. At the Hall I had been immersed in fear and thoughts about my illness, lifespan and death. Now my thoughts were focused outside myself, on the music, the singers and the elderly people.

There were about thirty female residents and two men. They were seated on high armchairs facing the front, except for one woman who was in a wheelchair. They, our audience, sat waiting for whatever would happen to them next, some with their heads lolling.

The members of 'Mirage' – Jaz, Dwight and Abi – were a startling sight. They were dressed in fire-engine red, sunshine orange and turquoise blue, and draped in electric-coloured scarves.

'This is how we fight back against institutional pastel decor', Dwight said, sweeping one hand vaguely towards his clothes, his gold chains and his silver earring. 'And the audiences love it.'

They opened the concert with a medley of sing-along songs, and my left hand rattled up and down the piano sketching in the harmony. Jaz stood in front of the audience while Dwight worked the room, occasionally taking a woman's hands and, as he sang to her, swinging them from side to side in time to the beat of the music.

A large woman with white hair fighting its way out of its bun was lolling back in a wheelchair with her swollen legs propped up in front of her. She had seemed to be asleep when we arrived, but now she began tapping her left hand on the arm of her wheelchair in time to the music.

'Why are you using only one hand?' Dwight was staring at the keyboard as I played the final chord.

'I've got no choice. I had an operation and my radial nerve was crushed accidentally. I can't operate my right arm or my hand.'

'Oh, poor you', he said. 'Bloody hard work.'

Jaz then announced 'Dwight is going to sing Harry Belafonte's song called *Island in the Sun.* Go for it, Dwight.'

Dwight launched into his song, and towards the end some of the audience joined in:

> I hope the day will never come
> That I can't awake to the sound of drum

Never let me miss carnival
With calypso songs philosophical.

Oh, island in the sun
Willed to me by my father's hand
All my days I will sing in praise
Of your forest, waters, your shining sand.

After every chorus Dwight and Abi did a kind of a jive that bore no relationship to the song's provenance. Jumping around in that residents' lounge where movement was usually slow and purely functional, they thrilled the audience with their sheer energy.

The woman in the wheelchair was joining in the singing, and when the others clapped, she banged her left hand on the arm of her wheelchair. I noticed that her right arm lay passively across her lap in a familiar position. Later, I walked over and asked her name.

She said 'Hello, dear. I'm Alice. You're a lovely pianist.'

'Well, I'm a one-handed pianist for the moment. My right hand is paralysed.' I pointed to it as it hung limp at my side.

'Get away! I never noticed.'

'Yes', I said. 'It was damaged in an operation, and I'm just hoping that it's going to come back again.'

'Don't worry if it doesn't, dear. You'll be all right. I can't move my right hand much either.' She bent her elbow and managed to move it about two inches off her lap. 'It's the arthritis. But I get by. There's always something going on here. And today's been a tonic.'

Back home I realised that, like Alice, I wasn't the same lethargic person that I had been earlier. Performing in the concert had energised me and pushed me out of the feeling of uselessness that was part of my 'ill patient' persona. I could still do some of the activities I used to do, even if I had to learn to do them in a different way.

My son, Lewis, made coffee while I sat with my right arm resting on the kitchen table. I thought about the residents in the old people's home. My illness and paralysed arm had shown me how difficult it is to go out and about when one is not 100% able, and that public space can be inhospitable to any but the completely fit.

Since my operation, shopping had turned into an obstacle course where I had to overcome the booby traps that the able-bodied placed in my way. Heavy fire doors impeded my entry to some shops. There was seldom anywhere to sit and rest. Shop assistants sometimes got impatient as they waited while I juggled my bag, purse and money one-handed.

Instead of assuming myself to be equal to whatever shopping challenge I might encounter, I had started to think of myself as a second-rate shopper who had to make that much more effort than a normal person in order to be taken seriously and achieve my shopping targets, whether it was to buy groceries in my local supermarket or to send a parcel at my local Post Office.

The residents in the old people's home had been livelier individuals by the end of the concert because they had been encouraged to sing and express themselves, whatever their handicaps. Were some of them there because the outside world expected them to be physically strong, to walk well, hear well and see well?

When I had returned from hospital and flicked through the fashion pages of a magazine, they had given me depressing intimations that I was part of what Morris in *Illness and Culture in the Postmodern Age* calls a 'culture dominated by the vision of utopian bodies.' According to this vision, not just my body but I myself could be seen as failing to meet its rigorous standards.

Morris links this kind of vision to the influence of biomedicine and its objective gaze – the one that I had feared from my first visit to the clinic, the gaze that can judge and categorise. It seemed that the power of this gaze had advanced outside the hospital, and it now became linked in my mind with the segregated residents in the old people's home.

Only now that I was scarred and disabled was I noticing how my community – the locality that I thought catered for locals – in reality only catered for healthy locals. When I had returned from hospital I had looked out of my kitchen window at people walking past and felt as if I were behind a glass screen. Now I realised that there were many other people behind glass screens, staring out at the world, needlessly cut off from everyday life by illness or disability.

A few days later, I woke up and saw the branches of the pine tree outside my bedroom window swaying in a sharp, late-summer wind. As I watched I automatically brushed the sheet against the fingers of my right hand and found that I could feel the drag of the cool cotton and its fine threads as I moved the material to and fro. My hand was coming back. Then I realised that I could bend my thumb a few degrees. I was ecstatic. This was just the beginning. By the end of the week I could bend my arm about ten degrees, arch my fingers and slightly wiggle my thumb. The whole process was awe-inspiring. Each day I could do a little more. What a pity my breast with its missing chunk of flesh could not be part of this process, but how magical that such an infinitely complex system as the hand and arm could regenerate itself after total paralysis.

Learning to be a patient was turning out to be like learning any other new role. Sometimes I was engrossed in its daily challenges, and other times I lost confidence and viewed myself only in relation to my imagination's perfect patient. When my paralysed hand and arm had upset the expected course of my cancer treatment, I had feared that I was a failing patient. Then I had learned that my fears were misplaced because my experience was not unusual. Countless others had entered hospital for a course of treatment only to have to adapt to detours – whether caused by side-effects, accidents or complications. Blood clots in the legs, wound infections, bedsores and other unexpected developments had challenged other patients just as my paralysed arm had challenged me. My side-effect was developing its own upbeat side-effect – a deeper sense of connection with others.

This gentle kind of learning and adaptation was disrupted by my arm's recovery. After the initial relief that my hand was getting back to normal, my thoughts turned inward again and I began to feel low. I had been practising *Solfeggietto in C Minor* by CPE Bach, as scored for left hand only, and I was due to play it in a concert the following month, but now I wondered what was the point. The rationale for the project would soon be gone and my right hand would be active again. I was relieved that my arm was recovering, but it meant that my priorities had to be worked out all over again. Furthermore, the sharp fear relating to my paralysis had distracted me from the dull, aching fear of my disease. I was left feeling confused, and nothing seemed worthwhile. Despite having numerous visitors, I was still alone for a large part of the day and found myself sinking into apathy. Everything had ground to a halt and I was yet again in limbo, just waiting to start the next round of treatment.

CHAPTER 14

One eye on the music

When I heard that a course called *Heal Your Life!* was running at the local Cancer Centre, I decided to give it a try. Julie was disapproving, just as she had been a few weeks previously about my visits to Bosom Friends.

'You don't need to go to the Cancer Centre. It's for people who are seriously ill. You don't want to start thinking of yourself as a cancer patient again. You've only just stopped being one.'

Part of me agreed with her and felt depressed at the prospect. But I was seeking something, anything that might inspire me and get me out of the rut of my apathy, and this might be it. My visit to the Bosom Friends support group had helped me and shown that the good patient is proactive and seeks help where possible. Why not seek help from another source of help for people in crisis, the self-help industry?

The course was based on the work of the American, Louise Hay, and in particular on her book *You Can Heal Your Life*. She was an international 'metaphysical' lecturer and writer who, her website proclaimed, had been dubbed 'the closest thing to a living saint' by the media. She had, it claimed, helped thousands of people to discover and use the full potential of their own creative powers for personal growth and self-healing. Jessie, the course leader, had been trained by another lecturer 'under the guidance' of Louise Hay. This tenuous global link-up was appealing to someone like me, who had been stuck in her own locality for such a long time. The course had already been running for two weeks, but the course leader agreed to take on a latecomer.

On a grey Thursday afternoon, Paul drove me over to a Victorian terraced house in the town centre. The founder, Eileen, greeted me and led me up the bare wooden stairs to a room on the first floor. Inside were seven women, sprawling on armchairs or sofas, obviously at ease with each other and laughing as we entered. Eileen introduced me to Jessie, the course leader, and the members of the group, all in their thirties and forties. I had applied to the course after it had started, and they had already spent two sessions together, but they welcomed me warmly, gatecrasher though I felt I was. Jesse moved a chair for me into the circle that they had formed.

'We always start off with a relaxation session', she explained.

Jessie was a trained hypnotherapist and had a voice that ranged from rasping to soft and soothing. She took us on a journey of visualisation up a mountain on a sunny day. I was soon absorbed in the vivid details of the winding mountain path, the lush green fields, the scarlet flowers and the singing floating upwards from a church down in the valley. Although in a trance, I was still aware of my surroundings, just as Jessie had promised.

When she brought us back into full consciousness I was amazed to find that the session had lasted 40 minutes, not the 10 minutes it felt like in retrospect.

Some of my deep relaxation ebbed away as we moved on to the rest of the agenda. I had missed the two previous sessions, which had been based on two affirmations – 'I am willing to change' and 'I deserve love, joy and all good.' Today we were going to work on developing awareness. Jessie talked about negative messages and about the importance of healing the inner child within each of us, and then asked us each to relate an experience in which our inner child had been harmed.

Despite being the newcomer, I was chosen to go first. I nervously related a tale about running away from home when I was about four years old. It was an event that I had rarely thought about in the past and had never shared with anyone before, but it darted sharply into my mind in answer to Jessie's question. I felt tense because I was afraid that I'd chosen an experience that was too trivial or too serious or that just failed to fit in with the sort of stories which the others would pluck from their past lives. But when they came to tell them, their stories ranged from sombre to funny, and I was reassured.

As a late arrival it was important that I fitted in with the others. We had all been treated for cancer within the last six months, we all faced the possibility of imminent death and we had all been changed by the experience. Our lives had been jolted out of their normal patterns and expectations. We looked back on our past differently because we were forced to see it in relation to the fact that we might not have a future. The other women on the course would have been plagued by new thoughts and questions similar to mine, and a product of the same catalyst – life-threatening illness. That was why we were all here together on the course, depending on Louise Hay and the answers that she had to offer us.

The meeting ended after Jessie had told us that the next week's session was to be about willingness to change.

Outside, fine rain was drifting from the grey sky, but I still felt the warm sunlight of my mountain walk glowing behind my eyes and through my whole body. The experience had been worthwhile, and I hoped to be a changed person by the tenth and final session of the course.

I never went back. Why? I was too tired when the next Thursday came. The energy for starting something new had left me. I was too tired to put myself on the line, to expose my intimate thoughts and emotions, to risk saying the wrong thing or revealing a wrong attitude. I felt different to the others. They were open, friendly and confident, whereas I was boring, proud, provincial and stuck in a rut. I was trapped inside a heavy lacquered cover – hard, shiny, reflecting people back to them. They were sincere, open and genuine – authentic.

Just as when, newly out of hospital, I had related my illness story to visitors, so now I could feel myself behaving, speaking and valuing as 'they' behave, speak and value. Soon after coming out of hospital, I had read a 'beginner's guide' to the work of the philosopher Heidegger and his theory of 'inauthenticity.' I had also read Heidegger's own description, in *On Time and Being*, of his theory as a way of living and a form of self-understanding that relates to the anonymous 'they.' By understanding the notion of inauthenticity and relating it to the new challenges that were facing me, I thought that I had begun to free myself to be 'authentic.' Alas, self-development, especially when it comes to the complexities of the great philosophers, is not so easy. It seemed to me that at the most, self-understanding and transformation are cumulative – forward, back (but not as far back as your original situation), forward, back a bit.

The *Heal Your Life!* course was designed to increase self-esteem and well-being, but both attributes have to be at a reasonable level to start with in order to survive the demanding nature of the course with its intimacies and self-revelations among strangers.

I was not up to it. It was a reflection of my self-absorption that I ever applied to go on such a course when it was already up and running. The clumsiness of my abrupt appearance and equally abrupt departure was a true reflection of the untidiness of my emotional state. Angst, angst, angst. I berated myself with these neurotic and confused thoughts. Yet throughout this depressing time post surgery, although my main plot was floundering, I never hit rock bottom, and looking back I can see that it was because my continuous identities, particularly as mother and musician, were like subplots that kept my spirits and self-esteem at a functional level. They were identities that required continuous action and produced continuous reaction from significant others – family and fellow musicians. They kept me afloat, but even they were not powerful enough to give me the confidence to return to the next session of the course.

There was also another barrier that prevented me from returning. I had learned that one of Louise Hay's basic beliefs was that 'we create every so-called "illness" in our body.' Maybe I should not have been shocked by this. It was after all only the logical consequence of her belief that we can heal ourselves – or was it? I had understood the term 'healing yourself' to mean that it is possible to bring about improvements in one's own mental and physical health through factors such as changing attitudes and diet, and exercising more.

To put the blame for the illness and the onus of recovery on each of us individual patients seemed unkind. What if I developed advanced breast cancer? Would it be my fault because I had created it? How did the other women on the course react to the pressure of being told that their recovery depended on their own efforts, and that if their cancer returned it would be due to their own failure?

Doctors are there to deal with the medical reality of illness. They can be grimly authoritarian in the way that they expect obedience from their patients, but they are willing to share the responsibility for their patient's treatment and possible recovery.

Louise Hay's patient must be obedient and adopt the requisite attitudes, diet, exercise programme and so on, but she must also take sole, lonely responsibility for having contracted her disease and for eventually defeating it. To defeat it she must become a new person. It all seemed a lonely business to me. Hay was not interested in my past or in my relationships with family, friends or colleagues.

Reading her book, *You Can Heal Your Life*, I found that Hay specifically defined the ways in which each individual had caused her particular illness – for example, cancer is the result of 'deep secret grief eating away at the self ...', and blackheads are 'small outbursts of anger ...'.

This approach seemed to play on the female patient's vulnerability and readiness to assume guilt. In order to survive I would have to transform myself into a new and different person without any reference to my everyday life and the way it had been affected by the uncertainties of illness and being a patient.

The medical reality of my illness, my personal history, my personal circumstances and the social environment in which I lived were immaterial to Hay. I was shaped by these influences, but Hay wanted me to ignore them and try to form a brand new identity. She was only interested in the personal – in the isolated individual. For all these reasons I disapproved of Louise Hay's theories, even disliked them.

Yet the following Thursday I thought of those women communicating with each other in that small room, and I envied them. They were learning about personal power, surely a worthy aim despite what I had thought were the limitations of Louise Hay's philosophy. Learning about our 'inner child' – a free spirit untouched by social oppression – gives us a glimpse of freedom and power. It gives us the opportunity to relate this to the material realities of our lives, and it opens and empowers us for the possibility of change.

I could even see how we might welcome the idea of self-blame for our disease, because it puts us back in control – life has not suddenly run amok. Our own actions have caused our situation. And the upside of the self-blame is the conception of the power of hope. Although we have cancer, we still have it in our power to make ourselves healthy, as in the admonition of Norman Cousins in *Anatomy of an Illness as Perceived by the Patient*: 'Don't deny the diagnosis; try to defy the verdict.'

I shared the aspirations of the women on the course for a healthier, more confident and self-aware future. And I envied their bonding. What is more, my brief experience of visualisation and affirmations had made me realise their potential and made me eager to read other self-help books.

Louise Hay did not completely measure up, but she had given me hope that there might be a book or a course out there that would perform the miracle for me – that would be tailor-made to make me happy and relaxed and make everything that had happened to me fall into place so that I could carry on with the rest of my life.

This was how, like so many other people who have experienced serious illness, I very quickly became obsessed with self-help books and self-help websites. Whole sections of self-help books had crept into my local book-shop and my local library at some time in my past without my ever notic-ing them. Now I was seduced by them.

What was I seeking from these books?

- I wanted to regain the zest for life that I had taken for granted before my illness. I felt apathetic, unable to concentrate, and I often avoided social events.
- I wanted to feel useful again and not just exist as a patient, yet I also wanted to be a 'good patient' and follow the example of the women at Bosom Friends by helping others.
- I was still unable to give up my superstitious belief that if I tried hard to be a 'good patient', and utilised all available sources of help, I would deserve to return to my old life.
- The books would be like a selfless confidante, reflecting and sharing my fears and worries and even offering solutions.

In the days before mobile phones, my position as a doctor's wife had been an official mini-job that involved taking phone messages from patients. Sometimes it had been impossible to gauge the gravity of the crisis by the voice of the caller. A patient in severe pain with a kidney stone might give a minimalist account of their symptoms, risking confusion and delayed diagnosis but leaving me marvelling at the courage and restraint of this 'good' patient who didn't want to 'bother' the doctor. Now I, too, was ren-dered proud and inarticulate when it came to my own health crisis, and it was to books and to Gaia that I turned for sustained, secret help.

Most of the self-help books for women shared the same inspiring mes-sage of change and transformation. Like Louise Hay, they seemed to view women as existing in a lonely world where self-grooming of the soul and unilateral action were paramount. They were the logical extension of the make-up and fashion strictures voiced by the beauty experts who visited Bosom Friends. Work on yourself, do all that we recommend and every-thing will be all right – you will be successful.

At the start of each book I would feel convinced that this was going to be the book that got me out of my torpor, and I would read it with enthu-siasm and recognition. A few days after finishing it, I would have forgot-ten most of what it said.

This forgetfulness was partly a result of my listlessness, but was also due to the contradictory nature of the books themselves. Their message was that you have a centre – a true fixed identity – that is the real, essential you, but that you must also change this 'you' in order to be happy. It was confusing.

Stephen Russell's *Barefoot Doctor's Handbook for the Urban Warrior* man-aged to be both more playful and more consistent, and it put me back in touch with my vision in the garden centre. Applying the principles of ancient Chinese Taoism, Russell says that you should 'lose the myth of who you are. You're simply nobody ... you're just atoms moving in the everything, child of the Tao, and everything is yours.' It was just like my vision, in which I was nobody and yet part of the universe. It bypassed Louise Hay's absorption with the need to examine and change oneself. For someone like me who was sometimes introspective and capable of believing my own myth as 'patient' – as someone at the centre of an illness drama – these were liberating words.

With the help of Gaia, I came across the *Thought for Today* website of the Brahma Kumaris World Spiritual University, an organisation that claims to help people to bring positive energy and deep personal values into their daily lives. I knew little about the university except for the fact that it had 5,000 centres in over 84 countries. Once again I – the patient stuck in her locality – was beguiled by the global nature of a self-help movement. I signed up to receive a *Thought for Today*, and the daily motivational messages became tiny beams of sunshine in my life. They had a life and immediacy that they wouldn't have had if I had read them in a book. Each one came winging through the vastness of cyberspace to arrive in my email account, fresh for that day and addressed personally to me:

> When my energy diminishes or I feel threatened and insecure, I pour love into every task and my energy and serenity are restored.

> Happiness is not a destination, it is a journey.
> It is not tomorrow, it is now.
> It is not dependency, it is a decision.
> Change your thoughts and you can change your world.

> Rest does not come with sleeping, it comes with waking. This is both an insight and an action of enlightenment. When we are enlightened we realise that real rest is possible only when we become free of illusions and we no longer struggle against life.

These messages were little lessons in how to give up being stuck in the past and how to abandon regrets for loss of health. They contradicted the claims of other self-help gurus like Louse Hay, and they had the same message as Stephen Russell's handbook, namely that happiness does not lie in focusing inward, but instead it is crucial to focus outward on what is happening in the present. Here was a positive philosophy in which I could have faith – except that at one and the same time it involved rejecting the opposite idea, the value of reassessing my past.

The self-help movement lacked the easy cohesiveness that I had hoped for, but its contradictions were not surprising considering that it is led by individualistic, charismatic personalities, and its belief system ranges globally over different religions and philosophies. I was finding inspiration in two apparently conflicting approaches – 'review your past and learn that you can change' versus 'live for the moment': that is, the introspection advocated by Louise Hay and others versus 'lose your ego and focus outward.' To my bewilderment, it seemed to me that both approaches were helpful and grounded in reality.

It gradually occurred to me that it wasn't necessary to choose one approach over the other. I felt a surge of creative relief as I realised that I could take both approaches on board. I found each of them meaningful. Why should I have to choose between them? Only some authoritarian and received logic buried deep within me had dictated that I should accept one and reject the other.

The symbiosis of these two seemingly contradictory approaches reminded me of the spiritual environment of the Welsh chapel that I had attended when I was little. The services in Bethania Chapel, in Cymmer Afan, were all conducted in the Welsh language. I couldn't understand all of it, but it had a direct line to my sense of divinity. For me, as a little girl, divinity was in the drama of the preacher's voice that swept from loud anger to whispering soulfulness as he gave his sermon. It was in the 'hwyl', in the passionate beauty of the four-part-harmony hymn singing, and it issued from the green and purple mountains that surrounded the valley.

God was all around me when I sang in a Gymanfa Ganu, a festival of Welsh hymn singing, when I was seven. I stood upstairs, up in the gallery with the other children, occasionally looking down on the rest of the congregation beneath us, but mostly engrossed in singing the tonic sol-fa notes from the hymn book that I was holding. God for me was music, nature, the Welsh language and the community.

After one hymn, the preacher gave a short talk. I sat looking at him, drilled in attentiveness even though I could understand little of what he was saying. The congregation began to laugh, and I suddenly realised that they were all looking at me. I felt my face burning and tears came into my eyes. Instead of being a normal member of the congregation, I was the focus of attention. Even the preacher was smiling at me.

As we walked home along the main street, its terraced houses clinging to the hillside, my Welsh-speaking father reassured me. The congregation had been laughing with me, not at me. He reminded me of what he had said to me as he gave me my hymn book before we set off for the Gymanfa.

'Now you must sing in time with the conductor's beat. You must have one eye on your music and one eye on Mr Jones, the conductor.'

I had been baffled. 'How can I do that? How can I have one eye on my music and the other eye on Mr Jones?'

I had looked down at my hymn book, then up into the distance and then back down at my book again. 'I can't do it. It's impossible.'

My father had laughed and said no more, but he had passed on this little exchange to the Reverend Hopkins, who had then passed it on to the entire congregation.

Even so, he expected me to think that the audience was not laughing at me.

I felt mortified, but mortification doesn't last long when you're young, and I had faith in my father.

The next Sunday I went to chapel as usual. I joined in the hymns with the rest of the congregation and listened rapt to the voice of the preacher. Yet something was different.

As usual I recited a verse from the Welsh Language Bible. Every child had to learn a verse to perform in chapel. The default verse for anyone who forgot to prepare one was 'Duw cariad Yw' – the shortest verse in the Bible. 'God is Love.'

On that particular Sunday, I had learned the first few lines of the twenty-third psalm, 'The Lord is my Shepherd':

> Yr Arglwydd yw fy mugail:
> Ni bydd eisiau arnaf ...

I faltered and looked around me. As I met the eyes of the congregation, I suddenly became aware that they might have their own thoughts about me – some friendly, some critical. My innocence was lost. I stumbled over the rest of the words and then sank back into my seat. I no longer felt the freedom that came from feeling merged unconditionally into a benign community.

Until then I had taken it for granted that everyone in the chapel respected everyone else. I had taken it for granted that the chapel elders who sat in the Big Seat, a wide bench seat that undulated around the pulpit, were there by some divine right. They would look up at the preacher and murmur noises of agreement with the content of his sermon – 'Ie' or 'Da iawn.' Now I wondered who decided who would sit in the Big Seat. Were they the oldest men? They had to be men, because there were no women in the Big Seat. Were they the ones who knew their Bible best? Who chose them and why?

The congregation no longer seemed a warm, spontaneous unit. I had taken everything in chapel for granted as if it was all preordained and eternal, but now a dramatic event – the sight and sound of the congregation looking at me and laughing – had made me aware that I was an individual entity in a complex organisation. I became dimly aware of the forces that choreographed what went on in the chapel – aware of traditions and rules, and of individuals and groups assessing events and making decisions.

It was a turning point, opening out my understanding of myself, my chapel and the workings of my social world. Without realising it at the time, I was learning a dual way of looking at things. My notion of myself as an integral member of a supportive chapel community was able to coexist with my recognition of the objectivity of the rules and the judgements within that community.

Now, as I sought some kind of help and comfort to guide me through the challenges of illness and post-illness, I was taking on board another kind of duality – the self-help movement's seemingly contradictory emphasis on developing as a person, and losing one's ego. They were both necessary – the two could coexist. It was indeed possible to have one eye on the conductor and one on the hymn book. Some people preferred one way of looking at things and others preferred a different way, but all looked at life in both ways.

The self-help books were giving me the same simple message as my paralysed arm: life is messy, but don't just accept it – welcome it. I didn't have to use reason to get through my illness. I could learn to love complexity. And somewhere between the conductor's beat and my hymn book, somewhere in the movement between them, there might even lie the meaning of my illness. So you need to keep one eye on the conductor and one eye on the music – so what if it's difficult? That's life and you go with the rhythm. You do your best in your own way and embrace all possibilities. There's no need to make constant judgements about your situation, yourself or anyone else.

CHAPTER 15

Outpatient

Radiotherapy requires faith. It is invisible, involves no cuts and no blood, and there's not a solitary medic in the room – just an outpatient, alone on the treatment couch surrounded by loud machinery.

After the long weeks in limbo since my operation, I was now willing myself to put my trust in my radiotherapy treatment, despite the fact that I knew little about it. 'Faith is taking the first step even when you don't see the whole staircase', said Martin Luther King Junior, and I was about to take my first step.

My hospital handbook had described the radiotherapy process but not how it worked, other than the fact that it killed cancer cells. In my attempts to find information from Gaia, I had searched the Internet with the term 'radiotherapy', not 'radiation', and initially missed out all the American sites that would eventually be my main source of information.

Yet the result of this confusion was not completely negative. 'Radiotherapy' is a British term – a composite word that includes the upbeat concept of healing, namely 'therapy.' It put a positive spin on my treatment and my expectations of it. When I came across the American term 'radiation', it conjured up bleak images of human folly, of wars like Hiroshima or the horrendous accident of Chernobyl, where unknown, deadly rays pervaded the bodies of helpless victims. These two different terms gave me a bilingual overview of my mystifying treatment.

My body was now to be newly assessed and manipulated by new and unknown staff within a new and strange environment – the radiotherapy unit at Hillcrest Hospital on the other side of the city. Used as I was to the beginnings and endings that had so far marked my path through treatment, I initially felt confident about going forward into a new regimen of treatment.

The radiographers at that first simulation session took X-rays in order to plan the total radiation dose and to figure out all the angles at which the X-ray beams should aim at my body. I listened as they carefully explained the procedure. They asked questions to check that I had understood, and were satisfied with my answers. But as it turned out, I retained little of what they had told me. When it came to the reality of having X-rays – whatever they were – beamed at my body, I was too panicky and too unsure whether I had made the right decision to remember anything.

A surgical operation is a dramatic but commonplace event that I had learned to trust. Although it involves slashed skin and flesh, bleeding and suturing, it is a familiar procedure. It is performed in a busy theatre by highly trained surgeons aided by many other medical staff, all of whom fit into a reassuring hierarchical order.

Compared with the craft of surgery with its elemental wetness and the physicality of the surgeon's hands, radiotherapy is an invisible art. It is dry, knifeless and metaphysical.

The radiographers were obviously intelligent, and had all completed degrees in radiotherapy, but the two who were running my simulation session looked very young, especially against the backdrop of their huge, clumsy machines. Who did they answer to? During the course of my treatment no one explained to me who was in charge of making the decisions about it. Was it a backroom radiotherapy guru, my oncologist or some other master of this mysterious art? I was never told, and it remained a mystery to me. In the course of my radiotherapy treatment I never came across the equivalent of my consultant surgeon – an acknowledged expert in the theory and practice of my treatment. I later learned of the existence of a consultant radiologist, a specialist in X-rays, but I never knew whether he or she had overseen my treatment or not.

Had I opted for a mastectomy, I wouldn't now need to submit myself to radiotherapy. Why had I turned down a straightforward surgical procedure for a treatment that was so unfathomable?

Then one small action, despite my initial shudder of distaste, served to reassure me. Martine, one of the radiographers, squinted at my chest and put a small tattoo on its midway point.

'This will give us a standard measurement to work from', she said.

I stared down as she marked the spot and, despite my qualms, found it reassuring that all those scientific measurements, all those mathematical calculations, were dependent on the solitary human hand that made a small blue mark on my flesh. It was a mark that was equidistant from the left smooth, healthy breast and the right scarred, mutilated one. I would walk away from this unit still bearing my tattooed dot but, unlike the tattooed number of a concentration camp inmate, its purpose was not to track me. It was a mark that related to the singular medical treatment of my individual body. It was essential for the success of all the sessions that I faced. As such, this little tattoo became my emblem of trust.

Paul offered to reschedule his morning surgery so that he could accompany me to my first radiotherapy session but, grateful though I was for his offer, it didn't seem a good idea. He was too busy – he would find the inevitable waiting unbearable and would sit thinking about all the things that he could be doing instead. In any case, as a doctor he would not be at ease sitting among all those patients.

Emma also offered to take me to Hillcrest Hospital. Having recently gone through the whole thing herself, she would know how she could help me and would understand her importance to me. So I gladly accepted her offer to drive me there. It was only eight months since I had ferried her to some of her sessions. Now she was escorting me to mine.

Within a year there would be another transfer of the baton, and I would be ferrying Mary, my neighbour, to hers.

Hillcrest Hospital was on the other side of the city, and Emma embarked on a different route to the one I'd expected. My own usual route to the hospital's locality had been developed over the years because it was near the school that Meg had attended. I managed to restrain myself from comparing Emma's route unfavourably with my own tried and tested one, even though I knew that it was the fastest and most efficient route possible. I was wrong. Over the coming weeks I was to find that Emma and the other four friends who took it in turns to drive me to the hospital each had their own favourite route across the city, and each was as quick and effective as mine.

The waiting area in the radiotherapy department was a vast, sprawling high-domed space. We sat in upholstered chairs and gazed upwards at the ceiling and its glass panels that allowed glimpses of sky. I had grown used to the narrow corridor with the low ceiling that was the waiting area for Parkside's breast cancer clinic. There I had come across other women from my local area, most of them mothers like me. Despite the deadly cause of our alliance, it had often seemed like my cosy peer group. In that small, enclosed space, illness had seemed containable. Here I had the feeling that illness might be boundless. Here there was not just the local and specific clientele of my Parkside clinic, but men, women and even children from distant areas of the Midlands, and a few of them were lying down, ashen-faced, in wheeled beds. 'The art of life lies in a constant readjustment to our surroundings', says Kakuza Okakura in *The Book of Tea*, and as a patient I was yet again adapting to new spaces and new people.

When I had chauffeured Emma here I had been healthy and therefore immune to the nuances of this place. I had sat in the waiting area sipping coffee, reading snippets in outdated women's magazines, and talking to patients and carers. Now I was party to the deep heart of the place and was about to find out what Emma had faced during her mysterious absences when I had sat waiting for her, content just to pass the time.

A nurse appeared and led me to a pine-shelved unit containing rows of small plywood boxes, each of which contained a radiotherapy gown. She handed me the contents of box 15. Inside a brown paper bag was a hospital gown. Dark blue with big splashes of red roses and a neckline edged in red cotton, the gown glowed in that pale, clinical environment, and I immediately started to bond with it. Care had gone into its design, and it was possible to open it and reveal either the left or the right side of the chest as necessary, and thus ensure maximum dignity.

This soft cotton garment was mine as long as my treatment lasted, and it was to become my safety blanket. Each time I arrived for a session it was waiting for me, and as soon as I put it on it transformed me from outsider to insider as far as the other patients were concerned.

Lying on the table in radiotherapy room 7, I started to feel panicky. How did I know that the radiographers had worked out their calculations accurately? Had they got the right dose? Did they have the optimum angle?

Instead of asking anything so specific as to appear insulting to the professionalism of the radiographers, I asked one of them a casual question.

'Will the radiotherapy leave the healthy part of my body alone?'

'I'm Hannah, the senior radiographer.'

A woman in her early thirties came and stood beside me and placed her long, capable fingers on my arm.

'Would you like to sit up for a few minutes so that I can tell you a bit more about what we're going to do?'

She showed me a diagram of my right breast and pointed out the way that the rays would be angled in order to avoid important parts such as ribs and lungs. The X-rays would 'sterilise' only the area left behind by the surgeon after he had removed the cancerous lump. Any remaining 'nasty' cells that might cause a recurrence of the tumour would be killed off, while my 'good' cells and the rest of the healthy me would be spared and come to no harm.

For many time-constrained medical professionals, this harsh but simple language of polarities and conflict – the war between good and bad – is a quick and graphic way of communicating with their patients.

When I had first come across this personification of my biological cells – my 'nasty' cancer cells and my 'good' healthy cells – I had looked to two books to help me understand why I disliked it so much. These were *Illness as Metaphor* by Susan Sontag and *Speak the Language of Healing* by Susan Kuner and colleagues. In her book, Sontag discusses the nature of this war imagery and the way that it marginalises and often alienates people with cancer. We are typically described as engaging in a 'combat' – we are 'soldiers' in a 'fight.' But using this symbolism relating to patients' empowerment, Sontag argues, undermines the struggles of people with cancer, as well as the effort to treat it. Claiming that a patient can defy illness by their will lays blame on the patient for the onset of cancer. It also lays blame on them for the onset of end-stage disease when a 'warrior' loses their hard-fought but ultimately fruitless battle. Sontag identifies the same conflict between empowerment and blame that I came across among the sources of self-help, and she paves the way for its conceptual and linguistic reinterpretation. There are many other metaphors, and many other ways of thinking and speaking about cancer.

After reading Sontag's book, I noticed how often we patients used a gentler kind of language even if it did sometimes still retain the notion of patient empowerment. Emma often referred to her cancer in terms of climbing a high mountain. In his memoir *It's Not About the Bike*, Lance Armstrong, top cyclist, chooses to adopt the non-violent metaphor of the Tour de France, the most important bicycle race in the world. He refers to physical setbacks during treatment as 'change orders' or 'project delays.' In the book he recalls how he switched oncologists after the first doctor he saw told him that he would hit him so hard with chemotherapy that he would virtually kill him. Armstrong, like Emma, chose images of hope and natural progress that were more inspiring than Hannah's unwittingly bleak description of my body as a war zone.

She undid the right flap of my gown as I lay on the table, and she then lifted my right arm and placed it in the cuff above my head. She adjusted my upper body beneath the red target beam that was coming down from the machine. I moved slightly in order to help her.

'Don't try to help me', Hannah said immediately. 'Just relax and leave it to me.'

I was now ready for the radiotherapy to begin. The last of the radiographers to leave the room pressed a button on the wall. Judging by the speed at which they left the room, none of them really had faith in the 'healthy cells will be spared' theory.

I was left alone in the silent room, an outpatient in a strange hospital. I had been an outpatient and an inpatient at Parkside Hospital, but always thought of myself as just a patient. Now I felt myself to be an 'outpatient' – an outsider on alien territory. A few warm tears trickled down my cheeks. A red light flashed on and a machine started up. The machine crept over me, whirring, hissing and falling silent. After a few minutes, Hannah came back into the room and swung the arc of the machine over to the other side before leaving me again. The sequence was repeated.

I was alone but for this hard, vast machinery built on supra-human lines. I had never thought that I would one day be having 'radiotherapy.' It was a word that I associated – thanks to childhood memories – with fear and doom. Radiotherapy was for mature, stoical people, not for me.

What had happened to that 'me' who had been the enthusiastic disciple of Russell's *Barefoot Doctor's Handbook for the Urban Warrior* and all those other books with their philosophical wisdom? Alas, their insights had yet to worm their way into my subconscious. The downside of any book about changing your life is that you can read it much faster than you can master its lessons and put them into practice, so that in a crisis like this, one of my most primitive reactions surfaced, namely self-pity.

'Self-pity is a mixture of self-love and anger' according to one self-help book. 'Self-pity is a device you use unconsciously to prevent yourself fully engaging in the present moment and moving on in your life' says the *Barefoot Doctor's Handbook for the Urban Warrior*. Part of me, even after months of treatment, still thought of myself as that special Welsh mother sprung from a race of healthy ancestors and innately deserving long-term health and even happiness. I was stuck in self-pity.

Then, in that dark lifeless room, words came floating into my mind to challenge me, words not of a self-help guru but of a poet, William Blake:

> He who binds to himself a Joy,
> Does the winged life destroy;

He who kisses the Joy as it flies,
Lives in Eternity's sunrise.

The delicate imagery lifted my spirits, and for a moment it was as if the invisible X-ray beams were rays of sunshine that were healing me in their warm light.

Back in the waiting room, Emma was still sitting in the same chair, and when she spotted me she smiled and waved. Seeing her, I felt tearful again. She looked so familiar and so reassuring.

When I told her about my tears, she said 'Don't worry. I felt the same when I started my chemo, and when I began my radiotherapy I went through it all again.'

It was a consolation. Radiotherapy might be less gruelling than chemotherapy, but this was my first post-op cancer treatment, just as chemo was hers. Both treatments are blatantly harmful to your body but, given your life-threatening cancer, their good effects outweigh the bad ones. 'What happens is best.' I remembered what Hannah had told me – that the success rate of radiotherapy has soared over the years due to the use of the simulator and a proper radio plan. Your faith and gratitude have to outweigh your fears.

It all became routine after a while. Enter the building, drop your card into the basket at reception, fetch your gown and wait to be called. If you arrived early you might get called early. The time of your next day's appointment was written on a card and left in the changing room with your clothes.

The drawback was that the system gave only around 24 hours' notice of your next appointment, so it was difficult to continue to work through your radiotherapy. I had been forced to ditch my college lecturing job, and sometimes wondered how my students were getting on. Although I had enjoyed my work, I found it difficult to imagine myself in such a public role ever again, and I was conscious of how much my daily concerns had shrivelled into the domestic and the personal.

By the third week of my radiotherapy, Paul was determined to accompany me to a session. When I returned from the changing room wearing my gown, he stared curiously at it. I noticed that another woman was wearing the identical garment and, seeing my gown through Paul's eyes, it became a barrier between us. It marked me out as a victim and made me into a different, de-feminised person – someone at the mercy of the system and required to wear the prescribed uniform. In that clinical environment I saw Paul as a doctor looking at me as a depersonalised being, one of those patients he had to contend with every day.

Of course, I can see now that the thoughts that I gave Paul were my own thoughts. They were the result of my low mood and the relentless threat to identity that illness brings. The sociologist Renée Lyons notes that even the most confident individuals look outward to others for support and validation:

> However, since illness and disability are seen as countering contemporary values such as prosperity, speed, independence, self-reliance and productivity, it is not surprising that individuals and their relationships struggle to adapt to this new life terrain ...

Yes, thanks to my illness I was a different person with a different lifestyle – slower, unproductive and dependent. I looked at Paul as I tried to guess at who I now was in his eyes, trying to work out the new dynamics of our relationship. Illness had disrupted my old assumptions about myself, my relationships and my place in the world.

I had been warned that I would get very tired as my treatment progressed, and sure enough, as early autumn gave way to winter and the days grew darker, I became lethargic.

Sometimes I would say 'I think I'll go and lie down for an hour. I'm feeling very tired.'

Whoever was around – Paul, one of the children or a friend – would turn to me and it was as if I could see my vulnerable patient identity reflected back to me in their eyes, validating my decision and giving me permission to be vulnerable.

Another common side-effect materialised – the skin on my breast turned livid pink and I started to have intense hot flushes as a result of the hormone drug I had been prescribed. Diverse effects radiating from diverse treatment, they all absorbed my mind as well as disrupting my body.

One day, as Emma parked her car outside my house, she said 'Do you realise that we've talked about nothing but breast cancer all the way home from hospital?'

I was surprised by her question.

I frowned at her and said 'But breast cancer is so fascinating.'

The following day we called in at the art gallery in the city centre where her paintings of Welsh medieval princes were on display in an exhibition. She introduced me to the director, Mark, and his assistant, and they discussed her paintings.

'By the way, thanks for working with that material last week.'

Mark explained to me, 'Emma went off and bought heaps of jewel-coloured fabric and then used it as background for the sculpture and jewellery exhibits. It was a lot of work, but it was worth it.' He pointed at the dramatic displays.

'I was able to buy it quite cheaply so it didn't cost the gallery much', Emma said. 'I wandered around loads of different stalls in the market and it's amazing what you can pick up.'

Listening to her, I was shocked by the way my own horizons had shrunk. I had forgotten that she had a life outside cancer, and forgotten that I too had once had one. It was as if everything to do with my cancer was in bold and expansively italicised print while the rest of my life was pale grey and upright.

Back at home, I changed out of the shoes I had worn to the hospital and put on the blue velvet slippers that I had worn during my stay in Parkside Hospital for surgery. I stared down at them. My hospital stay seemed just a short time ago, and the slippers conjured up a memory that was not unpleasant. In hospital I had lived on the edge, coping with pain, not knowing what was coming next, but determined to survive. Now that adrenalin and that immediacy had vanished and I didn't know what sort of patient I should be. Should I be following my original quest and striving to return to my pre-illness life? Or should I be just trying to get through the radiotherapy sessions?

By session 14 of the 17 sessions, the whole sequence had swung into a familiar rhythm. Put your card in the patient in-box, pick out your gown in its brown paper bag from box 15, change into it, then sit, wait and chat with a friend or fellow patient, and head for the radio room when your name and room number are called. Have a brief chat with the radiographers as they check your position and before they exit the room. Lie still while the machines whirr and clamber over you. Exit the room, return to your cubicle, pick up the card stating the time of the next day's appointment that is already lying on the cubicle seat, change back into your own clothes, put your gown into the paper bag and return them to box 15, and finally depart with your friend. This was a simple routine, but it still sometimes alarmed me because neither the radiotherapy nor any positive results of it were apparent.

I remembered what a friend who specialised in alternative therapies had told me before I went into hospital for my operation: 'I'll send you Reiki, and if you believe in it, you will receive it.'

Radiotherapy also needs faith, even though its benefits are scientifically proven.

The time was fast approaching when my hospital treatment would be over. Now I was haunted by the fact that I would never be clear of the threat of cancer. The fear surfaced a few days before my penultimate radiotherapy session, on the day when I visited Parkside Hospital for a routine appointment with my consultant. As I sat waiting to see him in that familiar narrow corridor, the anxiety that I had felt on that first visit when I waited for his diagnosis flooded over me.

Molly, a Breast Care nurse whom I'd never encountered before, called my name and ushered me into the consulting room.

In a voice that I associated with the soft, carefully modulated tones of the graduate of a counselling skills course, she explained that she would be sitting in on the consultation.

I sat down and glanced out of the window. The sky, unlike that on the day of my diagnosis, was not profoundly blue but mistily grey.

Before the consultant could speak, I asked him a question. I had intended to speak only after he had spoken, but anxiety had blotted out my deference to the usual consultation protocol.

'Can you tell me, doctor, does the hospital store the slides of patients' tumours?'

I was worried about my treatment becoming stuck in time. Medical advances were taking place all the time. Maybe at some stage, new research would indicate that I should have had chemotherapy or some other treatment, and the medical staff would then be able to check my slides, analyse them in the light of new information and save my life by giving me the latest treatment regime.

'Why do you want to know?'

'I just thought that they might turn out to be useful if new treatments came to light.'

The consultant peered at me over his half-moon gold spectacles before speaking. Then, from the tone of his voice and the rhythm of his speech, I could tell that he was giving me a full and sympathetic answer, but I was stressed out, tired and incapable of focusing on the words that fell from his lips.

When the consultation had ended, Molly invited me to follow her through a door into an anteroom.

I sat down reluctantly when she offered me a chair. It was practical medical information that I wanted, the kind that was outside her remit.

'Now, tell me – what's really bothering you?'

I was silent.

Molly said 'Would you like to come in for a counselling session? We could arrange one for next week some time if you'd like to come. I think you might find it helpful.'

'Er ... no. I'll be all right, thanks.'

Nothing would be gained from it. I wanted to know about scientific possibilities and advances in the outside medical world, not waste time focusing uselessly on my own concerns and obsessions. There was nothing to be gained from talking to her.

Had Molly been Carys, my former nurse and mentor, I would have reacted differently. I knew Carys. For some reason, doctors were more interchangeable than nurses when it came to my trust. Perhaps it was because the expertise of the specialist nurse was not as familiar to me or as well defined as that of the doctors. The doctor, unlike the nurses, was keyed into the latest scientific thinking, thanks to his medical journals, medical courses and doctor colleagues.

I saw it as layered knowledge. Despite all the professional help that Carys had given me, I was still influenced by the traditional notion that a nurse is lower down the ladder than a doctor, and therefore a less important source of help.

By the time I got home I was regretting having turned down the opportunity that Molly had offered. My instinctive reaction had been to think that she was patronising me by not taking my worries at face value, but now I realised that I had been wrong. She had wanted to help me. She had recognised that I was fighting against the prospect of living with uncertainty, of not knowing what the future held. I had been hoping that the consultant would tell me that I had nothing more to fear, or at least that in the future a scientific panacea would be discovered.

I was wrestling with the realisation that when it came to my cancer, closure was unattainable. That was what was really bothering me. And Molly had challenged me to recognise my fear and move on from it.

I never did take up Molly's offer of counselling, just as I had never gone back to the *Heal your Life!* course. This time it was different. I didn't feel like a failure for not cooperating fully with the help that was offered. Molly had helped me just by asking a crucial question that had led me to greater self-understanding. Experience was teaching me that there are sources of help out there, people who will help you in all kinds of ways, and they sometimes succeed even if you don't utilise all the help that they offer. I just hoped that professionals like Molly recognised the nebulous effect of what they offered and didn't measure their success purely in terms of how much patients like myself cooperated with them.

There was another factor that prodded me towards the future and shook my dependency on my hospital persona. It was the realisation that hardly anyone I knew could claim to be a non-patient. The media are continually promoting food scares and miracle health foods alike, putting us all in the position where we are responsible for our own health and to blame if we become ill as a result of following the 'wrong' lifestyle. In that respect we are all 'outpatients' now, either striving to achieve or maintain health, or feeling guilty if we're not doing so.

Moreover, several of my friends had acute conditions that waxed and waned, or had chronic ailments that hung on, like diabetes, chronic arthritis and coronary heart disease.

After a friend's unexpected fatal heart attack, it occurred to me for the first time that some other serious illness could befall me. I had come to see myself through the doctors' eyes as a cancer patient, someone under their control, along with my body and its health. In fact my body was individual and therefore open in its individualistic way to any number of new afflictions. The threats of cancer had not reduced the chances that I could develop another serious illness or even some other kind of cancer. Illness does not distribute itself fairly and equally. Nature is random and, despite the advances of medical science and however closely I was monitored, I was still at its mercy.

At the sixteenth radiotherapy session my routine was disrupted. I had an appointment to see a physician, and sank down into an armchair in the waiting room after my session was over. In the quiet corner opposite me a pale, skinny little boy was lying on a hospital trolley. He had a tube leading from his fragile arm to the small bag of colourless fluid attached to the drip stand. Despite all the new treatments and new medicines that had been developed since my own childhood, this little boy was still suffering. When I was a child, I had assumed that I was immune to illness and death. This poor little boy had lost the childhood trust and innocence that were his by right. He had learned that adults can be helpless and that children can suffer.

A young woman with an angry, angular tattoo on each upper arm stood next to his trolley, staring into space. When the little boy started to fiddle with the cannula that was protruding from his hand, she stepped across, leaned over him and slowly swept a strand of fair hair from his eyes. His hands relaxed by his side and he smiled at her with such trust that I realised that this was his carer, possibly his mother, and I was wrong about his lost innocence.

If I was wrong about this, what other events and experiences – my own and those of others – had I misinterpreted during my illness? In this case, I had failed to foresee the resilience of a child's trust, possibly because of my own crisis of faith in the future. I realised yet again that what I was seeing was through my own eyes and my own preconceptions, and not through some generic patient's eyes. This being so, how could I aspire to be some mythical 'good patient'? Yes, I could aspire to be a good patient, but only through my own idiosyncratic eyes.

A nurse emerged from the door immediately opposite my chair and ushered me into the consulting room. She asked me to remove my upper-body clothing and lie on the examination couch, and she then covered my body with a blanket. The doctor entered, spoke only to check my name, and lowered the blanket to reveal my overheated breast with its livid red scar.

No sooner had he done so than the door opened, and I could hear the voice of a secretary asking him a question about a letter. I couldn't see her because I was lying facing away from the door. The doctor answered her, and they then embarked on a lengthy chat about a nurse who was off sick. The nurse walked over and shut the open door that left me visible to passers-by, while the doctor and the intruder stood above me, carrying on their casual conversation. I pulled the blanket up to my chin. After moving between me and the woman in order to block her view, the nurse patted my shoulder. Our eyes met and she sighed, 'Oh, bad.'

After a brief look at my radiated chest, the doctor wrote out a prescription for an emollient cream. He was the only physician I had seen at Hillcrest Hospital, and I had expected him, like the other doctors who had examined me during the course of my treatment, to show that he knew my medical history and to ask me how I was feeling. Instead, with practised finality, he handed over my prescription. The consultation was over.

To this doctor I seemed to be composed of non-cohesive bits and pieces – an operation and some radiotherapy sessions here, a sore area of skin there – just an anonymous outpatient shifting in and out of medical view.

Once I was outside in the waiting room again, I felt upset by the way my consultation had been turned into a social encounter between the doctor and the secretary. I was also annoyed with myself. By now my former amenable patient persona should have developed into a confident assertive one. I should have complained instead of just lying there passively. How could I have been so pathetic? But then I began to see my faintheartedness in perspective. Patients are always having to react rather than act. In the course of reacting, I had done the best I could given the circumstances.

- Countless other women had reacted in the same way after suffering similar indignities to mine. I had heard their stories during visits to meetings of Bosom Friends.
- All we patients are to a certain extent inured to this hierarchical system in which the doctor is top of the heap.
- Not even the nurse had dared to confront the doctor, even though she resented his behaviour. Admittedly the nurse was in the system and her job might be on the line. Admittedly it would have been more effective for me, as a patient, to complain. But, as a patient, I felt vulnerable and tired.
- The doctor was a stranger to me. It was best to be cautious.
- I was still making progress as a patient. The fact that I was finishing my hospital treatment didn't mean that my progress as a patient was over and this was the best patient I would ever be.

Walking along the corridor I met Hannah, the senior radiographer, and grumbled about the idle conversation that had been conducted over my prone body.

'Unprofessional behaviour to say the least. I'm sorry about that.' Hannah sounded sympathetic but unsurprised.

She led me over to the radiographers' office.

'I'm glad you've agreed to put in a complaint. Complaints really do work around here. They take notice of what patients think.'

She handed me a complaints form.

'It's your final session tomorrow, isn't it? How did you find the treatment? Lots of patients find radiotherapy difficult – they find it difficult to put their faith in it.'

I hadn't realised that my fears were so commonplace.

'My faith came and went, but mostly came ... and I'm very grateful for the treatment.'

Yes, I had found it difficult to have faith in my radiotherapy treatment. In fact it had been an ongoing struggle but, over time, fear had mostly been overtaken by wonder at this mysterious, life-prolonging treatment. Faith had been a process rather than a way of thinking – as the writer, Edith Hamilton, has identified: 'Faith is not belief. Belief is passive. Faith is active,' Although I still knew nothing about the science of radiotherapy, I had learned what I needed to learn in order to have a measure of faith in it.

CHAPTER 16

Understanding

It was now six months since that sunny June day when my consultant had stunned me with his cancer diagnosis. On the day after that momentous hospital visit, I had visited historic Middleton Hall, and it was there that I had first faced the fears that led me to make my short-term and humble pact with fate. I would live the life of a good patient so that at the end of my hospital treatment I would still be unchanged and would return to my old familiar life. I would work my way towards the end of illness and arrive at closure. I would no longer be a patient. My old life would resume.

Now I was about to complete my final session of radiotherapy. It marked the end of my six-month schedule of treatment, but now it turned out that the closure I had counted on was not an option. I was still swallowing the pills for my hormonal treatment. I would still have to attend the hospital for check-ups, and there was no one who could tell me that my cancer was cured. I was unable to be that good patient who reached the end of her hospital treatment and put it all behind her, end of story. Now I had to live with uncertainty.

Yet it was not so bad. Being a patient, it now seemed to me, was like being a mother or being Welsh. It was a role that came and went, but would always be part of my identity. I no longer reacted with dismay when friends or acquaintances related to me as a patient. I no longer thought that they were classifying me as a one-dimensional inferior being, and I believed it was quite possible that they were respecting my humanity and vulnerability.

Looking back, I saw my successes and failures as a patient as a kind of normality. The word 'patient' now had rich connotations for me – fear and affliction, yes, but also opportunity and freedom. Six months of medical crisis and treatment had forced me to move into a different world so that what I had thought of in my old world as fixed turned out to be just one way of doing things, just like the route of my journey to radiotherapy, where I had thought that mine was the only effective route.

As a child singing in a Gymanfa Ganu, I had pondered over the paradox of singing with one eye on the conductor and one eye on the hymn book. Now, as an adult, I was facing the nature of this paradox and learning, in a raggedy kind of way, to give up some of my old assumptions and to live with complexity, change and contradictions. I had been given the opportunity to step outside my life and to see its strengths and its constraints – the self-imposed constraints as well as those imposed by outside forces.

Now I understood why Samira Khan, the woman in Rushwood Hospital, had said all those months ago that cancer was the best thing that had happened to her. At the time I had been embarrassed by such a weirdly sentimental comment, but after six months of unsteady progression through the ongoing challenges of illness I knew what Samira meant.

She would naturally give anything not to have cancer, not to be ill and not to live with the threat of death, but having a life-threatening illness gives a woman a certain freedom. It allows her to try on different personas. She frees herself from some of the usual social constraints because she sees herself as a patient, humble but also different and deserving. Others often look at her with soft, approving eyes rather than the cold, appraising ones of her female imagination. She may, perhaps for the first time ever, feel free to work out her own personal priorities.

My quest to be a good patient had been a game, but it had been a serious game. It had raised ethical questions.

'What is a good patient?'

'What should you do, how should you act and how should you be in order to live as a good patient?'

And I had found that those questions were inseparable from my relationships with people and places.

- The 'good patient' – in whose eyes? Would they be those of my family, the hospital staff, my fellow patients or myself?
- The 'good patient' – in which place? Would it be the clinic, the ward, the home, the support group meeting or the deserted radiotherapy room?

My quest hadn't had the outcome that I had originally sought, but the questions that it raised had given meaning to my treatment and had given me the opportunity to define myself instead of being defined only by the medical professionals and by my disease. It had given me a degree of control over all the shifting circumstances triggered by my illness.

Had I won my self-invented game, the fates would have allowed me to remain the same person as before my illness. I had lost, but I was a graceful loser because I had accepted that my quest had been based on a fallacy. I had thought that even though my body was being changed by illness, my identity could remain static and 'fixed.' But illness is a mind–body experience and relentlessly brings changes to one's identity as well as to one's body. Thanks to my own experiences, and thanks to Emma, the women at Bosom Friends, Gaia and all the insights from writers and theorists, I was now recognising that illness was not an interruption to my life but an integral part of it. This knowledge had not come easily, but a new patient is brought back time and again because they don't catch on the first time, and life brings them back for another glance at the situation, from a slightly different angle.

The good patient learns to accept and adapt to the many challenges that illness presents to their old identities. And there lay the answer to the question that had threaded through the period of my treatment: 'What is a good patient?' The answer was not really an answer at all – more an art or a style of living – and as a statement it was so spare that it seemed platitudinous. But no one could say that it was easy: 'The good patient learns to surrender to the rhythm of life.' It's best neither to struggle against it nor to endure it passively, but rather to summon up a spirit of adventure in order to embrace it. In the secret life of a patient, random and sometimes chaotic things happen that are rarely reflected in the simple linear progress of the medical records. There is a secret ebb and flow to faith and doubt, trust and suspicion, the simple and the complex, courage and fear, empathy and indifference. It is in these apparent contradictions that the meaning of life is found, meaning that Eliot vividly evokes in the second of his Four Quartets – East Coker: 'So the darkness shall be the light, and the stillness the dancing.'

These days, when I look back at the six months of my treatment, I sometimes glimpse again those two mystic visions, one in the consulting room and the other in the garden centre, visions that filled me with an awesome sense of communion with others. They were signs of that mysterious abundance that illness can unveil. Then those familiar gentle words from my childhood come back into my mind: 'What happens is for the best.' It is strange to think that I once thought my grandmother's words simplistic.

On this, my seventeenth and final visit to Hillcrest Hospital, I took a camera and asked Martine, one of the radiographers, to take a photo of me with the other radiographers. I think I was trying to force them to appreciate the significance of my personal milestone. After that, my sojourn as a hospital patient would be over. In the coming week, I would be returning to my job as a lecturer at my local college. In the snapshot I pose tensely between two cooperative and politely smiling radiographers. There we stand awkwardly, caught in a time that was ending. For them I was just another patient, but to me they were my link with a momentous time in my life. Behind us looms the vast machine that had radiated my body a few moments earlier.

Part of me welcomed the end of my treatment, because I was tired of it and wanted to move on to a new stage. But another part of me saw myself as the patient depicted in my medical notes, the one who was a pawn of the doctors and whose life was simple and dictated by the medical treatment. There was a fear in contemplating the wider world without that familiar 'patient' persona.

My life had been rooted in the two hospitals and my home, but now I would have to go out into other spaces and mix with people who knew nothing of my medical history. I had learned to rely on my identity as a member of a minority group with an obvious wound. Now I had to go back to being an 'ordinary' person whose strengths, weaknesses and idio-syncrasies are hidden.

Except that now I felt less pressure to be always successful and smooth. What happens is for the best. My 'patient' persona had helped me to reveal myself to others – strengths, weaknesses and all – and now that I would no longer be defined by it, maybe I didn't need my old defensive persona back either, that lacquered shell that had once separated me from others.

As I headed towards the changing cubicle for the last time, I passed another woman on her way into Room 5. She seemed to be new – I had-n't seen her before. She hesitated, stared and gave me a one-sided smile. As she moved on I noticed, just visible under the collar of her coat, the scarlet neckline of a gown like mine. If only I had noticed it sooner, I would have spoken to her.

And so it went on, the endless march of women in and out of Room 5. Only a few months later I would be back with a friend. I would once again bear vigil in the waiting area, flick through a similar pile of ancient mag-azines, talk to a brand new group of patients, friends and relatives. My friend would wear the identical scarlet-patterned gown, that soft cotton token of solidarity and shared suffering. She would face the same fears and be left with the same loneliness in the deserted radiotherapy room. She might even come to view her gown as a kind of comfort blanket, just as I had once done, although now I knew that its comfort would always be with me even when its soft touch was nothing but a memory.

I came out of the cubicle, put my gown into its paper bag and started walking past the reception area towards the shelves to put it back into box 15, but Liz, the receptionist, leaned over and stretched her arm out.

'No need to put it back – you've finished your treatment.' Liz smiled at me and lifted it gently out of my hands.

'You won't be needing this any more.'

Afterword

Here, high on the mountain, there is a chilly sense of vast space. Dark shapes loom and the yodel of a herring gull echoes way above. Spurred on by my daughters, Meg and Ceri, I have climbed up to the summit of Snowdon just one day after my fifth and final annual check-up. I sit and rest on a small ridge after the tough scramble to the top and feel cold rock beneath my hand – rock worn smooth by the steps of countless others who have lingered here on the heights, and looked back down on the arduous slopes.

The peak is covered in mist and, although I can feel its timeless beauty, I can't see the view clearly so I don't know exactly what's ahead. But do any of us know? Like me, our fellow climbers here on the summit just seem exhilarated to have made it to the top. I look at them, newly aware that there will be people like me among them – people whom Susan Sontag describes as living with a visa, living in the land of the healthy while still not wholly or permanently so themselves.

As I look over to the vast unseen spaces across the deep valley, images come to mind of my friend and guide, Emma, who died two years ago following the recurrence of her breast cancer, just three weeks after running her last art workshop in Aberystwyth. I think of Samira Khan, my first friend in illness, of the active members of Bosom Friends and the many other women like them who, as a result of leading what Audre Lord calls 'a considered life', commit time to causes such as healing, charity or health politics.

Each had to work out for herself how to be a patient, and each struggled to find meaning in her illness, just as I and so many other women have done. In the course of time, we learned from others' actions and stories, and somewhere in the extended process we gained the 'boon' of illness – what Bruner describes as 'the ability to mourn and to rejoice not for yourself only but for others. To lose the secrecy and fear.'

Now, on this cool summer day, the sublime sense of all this is out there in the boundless spaces of Snowdonia. It is out there, hidden in the mists, the elusive nature of universal love.

Soon it is time to begin our descent of Snowdon and return to base. As we are about to leave, the mist recedes for a moment and I glimpse the blue sky that embraces the stark contours of the mountain.

Further reading

Adamson J, Freadman R and Parker D (eds). *Renegotiating Ethics in Literature, Philosophy and Theory.* Cambridge: Cambridge University Press; 1998.

Armstrong L. *It's Not About the Bike: my journey back to life.* London: Yellow Jersey Press; 2001.

Blake W. *The Complete Poems.* Harmondsworth: Penguin; 1978.

Bolen JS. *Close to the Bone.* New York: Scribner; 1996.

Brahma Kumaris. *Thought for Today.* World Spiritual Organization; www.brahmakumaris.org.uk/thought/tft.asp

Braidotti R. Nomadic subjects: embodiment and sexual difference in contemporary feminist theory. In: Eagleton M, editor. *Feminist Literary Theory.* Oxford: Blackwell; 1995.

Brody H. *Stories of Sickness.* Oxford: Oxford University Press; 2003.

Broyard A. *Intoxicated by my Illness.* New York: Fawcett Columbine; 1992.

Bruner J. Self-making and world-making. In: Brockmeier J, Carbaugh D, editors. *Narrative and Identity.* Amsterdam: John Benjamins; 2001.

Butler J. *Gender Trouble: feminism and the subversion of identity.* London: Routledge; 1990.

Christakis N. *A Death Foretold: prophecy and prognosis in medical care.* Chicago: University of Chicago Press; 1999.

Couser GT. *Recovering Bodies: illness, disability and life writing.* Madison, WI: University of Wisconsin Press; 1997.

Cousins N. *Anatomy of an Illness as Perceived by the Patient.* New York: WW Norton; 1979.

Duff K. *The Alchemy of Illness.* New York: Random House Inc.; 1993.

Eliot TS. *Four Quartets.* London: Faber and Faber; 2001.

Forster EM. *A Passage to India.* Harmondsworth: Penguin; 2005.

Forster EM. *Howards End.* Harmondworth: Penguin; 2000.

Fosket J. Problematising biomedicine. In: Potts LK, editor. *Ideologies of Breast Cancer.* Basingstoke: Macmillan Press; 2000.

Foucault M. *Health and Medicine.* London: Routledge; 1997.

Foucault M. *The Birth of the Clinic* (translated by Sheridan AM). London: Routledge; 1986.

Frank AW. *At the Will of the Body: reflections on illness.* Boston, MA: Houghton Mifflin Company; 1991.

Frank AW. *The Wounded Storyteller.* Chicago: University of Chicago Press; 1995.

Freeman M and Brockmeier J. Narrative integrity. In: J Brockmeier and D Carbaugh (eds) *Narrative and Identity*. Amsterdam/Philadelphia: John Bejamins; 2001:75.

Fulghum R. *From Beginning to End: the rituals of our lives.* New York: Ballantine Books; 1995.

Gill S, editor. *Selected Poems of William Wordsworth.* Harmondsworth: Penguin; 2004.

Grimes RL. *Deeply into the Bone: re-inventing rites of passage.* Berkeley, CA: University of California Press; 2002.

Hamilton E. *Witness to the Truth.* New York: Norton; 1962.

Hay L. *You Can Heal Your Life.* Enfield: Eden Grove Editions; 1987.

Heidegger M. *On Time and Being* (translated by Stambaugh J). Chicago: University of Chicago Press; 2002.

Hertz R, editor. *Reflexivity and Voice*. Thousand Oaks, CA: Sage Publications; 1997.

Illich I. *Limits to Medicine*. London: Marion Boyars Publishers Ltd; 1976.

Kafka F. *The Penal Colony: stories and short pieces* (translated by Muir W and Muir E). New York: Schocken Books; 1948.

Kenyon J. *Collected Poems*. St Paul, MN: Graywolf Press; 2005.

Kleinman A. *The Illness Narratives: suffering, healing and the human condition*. New York: Basic Books Inc.; 1988.

Kuner S, Orsborn CM, Quigley L and Stroup KL. *Speak the Language of Healing*. Nashville, TN: Conari Press; 1999.

Lorde A. The cancer journals. In: *The Audre Lorde Compendium*. London: Pandora; 1996.

Lyons RF, Ritvo PG. *Relationships in Chronic Illness and Disability*. London: Sage Publications; 1995.

McAdams DP. *The Stories We Live By*. New York: Guildford Press, 1993.

Miller H. *Stories, Essays, Travel Sketches*. New York: MJF Books; 1992.

Morris DB. *Illness and Culture in the Postmodern Age*. Berkeley, CA: University of California Press; 2000.

Moss P, Dyck I. *Women, Body, Illness: space and identity in the everyday lives of women with chronic illness*. Lanham, MD: Rowman & Littlefield Publishers Inc.; 2002.

Murphy RF. *The Body Silent*. London: WW Norton & Company Ltd; 1990.

Okakura K. *The Book of Tea*. New York: Dover Publications; 1964.

Parsons T. *The Social System*. Glencoe, IL: Free Press; 1951.

Potts LK, editor. *Ideologies of Breast Cancer: feminist perspectives*. Basingstoke: Macmillan Press; 2000.

Reed-Danahay DE, editor. *Auto/Ethnography*. Oxford: Berg; 1997.

Russell S. *Barefoot Doctor's Handbook for the Urban Warrior: a spiritual guide*. London: Judy Piatkus; 1998.

Sacks O. *A Leg to Stand On*. New York: Summit Books; 1984.

Schneider CE. *The Practice of Autonomy*. Oxford: Oxford University Press; 1998.

Sherwin S. *No Longer Patient: feminist ethics and health care*. Philadelphia, PA: Temple University Press; 1992.

Sontag S. *Illness as Metaphor*. New York: Farrar, Straus and Giroux; 1978.

Stacey J. *Teratologies: a cultural study of cancer*. London: Routledge; 1997.

Strauss AL. *Mirrors and Masks: the search for identity*. London: Martin Robertson; 1977.

Van Gennep A. *The Rites Of Passage*. Chicago: University of Chicago Press; 1960.

Watts M. *Heidegger: A Beginner's Guide*. London: Hodder and Stoughton; 2001.